Dedicatic

Anne Smeijsters

Eric Clapton

Acknowledgments

Barcelona Publishers gratefully acknowledges the permission to reprint the following chapters granted by various people and organizations: CRP-Santé Luxembourg Fonds National De La Recherche for Chapter 1, Musiktherapeutische Umschau for Chapter 2, University Witten-Herdecke for Chapter 3, Nordic Journal of Music Therapy for Chapter 6.

The author would like to thank all colleagues who by their writings and discussion helped him to develop the theory of analogy. Special thanks to Carolyn Kenny who inspired the author to keep in touch with the client's and the music therapist's experience.

CONTENTS

Foreword *ix*
Introduction *xi*

PART I: RESEARCH AND THEORY IN MUSIC THERAPY

Chapter One

Multiple perspectives on the development of an evidence-based music therapy: A personal history 3
Introduction 3
The development of research topics in music therapy 4
The agenda for the future: Peer debriefing 14

Chapter Two

Criteria for indications in music therapy 15
Introduction 15
Research 16
Examples of indications 21
Discussion 28
Epilogue: A client-focused and evidence-based music therapy treatment 29

Chapter Three

Toward a general theory of music therapy? 31
Introduction 31
The dialogue 31
Peer debriefing 36
A categorization of questions and statements 38

PART II: TOWARD A THEORY OF ANALOGY IN MUSIC THERAPY

Chapter Four

The power of music 43
Introduction 43

Form and content 43
Cognitive processing 44
Music: The irrational and numinous 45
Referential meaning of 'empty' words 46
Symbolic knowledge 48
Intimate knowledge 50
Conclusions and outlook 52

Chapter Five

Analogy: A core category in the writings of music therapists 55
Introduction 55
Research 56
Examples of concepts used by music therapists 59
Analogy as a core category 60
Epilogue: Triangulation 63

Chapter Six

Forms of feeling and forms of perception 65
Introduction 65
To begin with: The hypothesis and one example 66
A perspective from psychology 67
A perspective from art 81
Therapy beyond words: Personal change by analogous experiences 83

Chapter Seven

Defining and redefining the core category of analogy 87
Introduction 87
Defining analogy 87
A glossary of concepts 91
Objections 100
Toward an intermediary language 101
A semiotic perspective from music therapy clinical practice 104
Epilogue: Redefining analogy 109

Chapter Eight

The analogy of musical interaction and the development of an independent self 111
Introduction 111

Theme and variation between mother and child 113
Conservation and variation in music and music therapy 117
Epilogue: The analogous triangle 134

Chapter Nine

Examples of analogy from research and clinical practice 135
Introduction 135
The man who could not drive his car 136
The woman who struggled with her mother 138
A fight between mother and daughter 139
The woman who locked herself in a cage 141
The man who passed the 'point of no return' 143
The man who lost his future 145
The girl who was not there 150

Chapter Ten

Researching analogies 153
Introduction 153
Knowledge development by triangulating clinical experience, naturalistic inquiry, and double-loop learning 155
Principles of naturalistic inquiry 161
Techniques of naturalistic inquiry 163
Naturalistic inquiry on analogies 168
Epilogue 180

Chapter Eleven

Epilogue: A never-ending story 181
Analogy 182
Metaphors, symbols and signs 183
Musical meaning 183
Verbal language 184
Expression and impression 185
Closing 186

References *187*
Index *205*
The Author *215*

FOREWORD

> *"Can you describe your experience in Music Therapy to me?" I said.*
>
> *"Well, it's subtle," she said. "I think of it like a needle and thread. In the music I can begin to slowly sew the fragmented parts of myself into someone whole."*

This is a conversational fragment from a talk I had with my music therapy client the other day. A great deal of the treatment, in this case, has been musical improvisation at the piano.

So often we hear descriptions of music therapy that contain the term "like." How many times have we heard the adage, "Music begins where words end?" This makes it rather ineffable.

We don't want to lose the unique characteristics of music and music therapy in our descriptions. But we have to use words to describe our experiences and to move toward understanding them.

In *Sounding the Self: Analogy in Improvisational Music Therapy*, Henk Smeijsters attempts to come to terms with the many paradoxes contained in our efforts to describe our work in music therapy improvisation. He has chosen analogy as the bridge between the music and words. He offers us a thorough elaboration of the concept of analogy and describes why this concept might serve as the center of a theory for music therapy. And he provides many examples to show us how analogy works its way through Music Therapy practice. Smeijsters' book is based on some of the best research available to music therapists around the world.

When I first met Henk Smeijsters, we were presenting research at the first Qualitative Research Music Therapy Symposium in Düsseldorf, Germany in 1994. At the time, I recognized a scholar and researcher experienced in the quantitative traditions, but who was seriously questioning the ability of a purely quantitative research approach to document the capacity of music therapy research to consider the full range of clinical work. Subsequently, we joined our efforts to consider the possibility for a general theory for music therapy and presented our work together at the 4th European Conference of Music Therapy in Leuven, 1998.

Since that time, I have watched his steady gathering of colleagues to discuss music therapy research and theory. In his new book, this spirit of collaboration is a guiding force.

It may be that analogy and metaphor offer us the best possible means to describe and even understand certain processes in music and music therapy. But analogy and metaphor pull us into literary forms. Music therapists often work in medical settings that demand evidence-based results from our research. In a very original and creative way, Smeijsters manages to bring the worlds of art and science together creating another bridge for debate and discussion. He leaves no stone unturned and his penchant for critical analysis will serve the music therapy profession well. He considers the multidisciplinary and interdisciplinary implications of his theory of analogy for creative arts therapies and developmental and cognitive psychology. This is a rich territory to explore in which Music Therapy will not be the only beneficiary.

I hope that you will enjoy the propositions, the questions, the examples, and the complexities of Smeijsters' work. His ideas will bring us into an understanding of some of the depth experiences in Music Therapy—the ones most difficult to describe in words.

Carolyn Kenny
Institute for Social, Behavioral, and Economic Research
University of California
Santa Barbara, California
USA Introduction

INTRODUCTION

This book gives a complete overview of the theory of analogy, which has been developed in the last decade. Until now, I had presented and published several theoretical and research papers independently in journals and during congresses, but there was not a complete overview in which all aspects were integrated. With this book, I fulfilled a personal wish and, since other authors have referred to the theory of analogy as an important contribution to the theory of music therapy, I hope that it will satisfy those colleagues who want to use this theory in clinical practice and develop it further.

The book consists of two parts. The first part has a more general character and paves the way for the second part, which focuses exclusively on the theory of analogy.

The books starts with a chapter that gives an impression of research topics that have been developed during the 20 years in which I have been researching music therapy (Chapter One). Today, some of the topics seem to be less important, but other topics are as important as never before. They will return in the chapters of the book.

In Chapter Two, the peer debriefing study about indications is described. By this study, I tried to find an answer to the question, "How can we know which treatment is appropriate for the client?" This research resulted in a set of questions a music therapist should try to answer to make sure that his music therapy method leads to treatment goals that increase the client's health.

In Chapter Three, a peer debriefing study about the possibility to develop a general theory of music therapy is described. When I started developing the theory of analogy, I had questions about music therapy in general, which I shared and discussed with several colleagues all over the world. Listening to the arguments of competent colleagues makes you modest. A researcher should be modest when developing theory because there is not just one theory of music therapy. The multiple, rich, and complex perspectives of people who are involved with music therapy should not be reduced to one single set of concepts.

The second part on analogy starts with a philosophical chapter on knowledge (Chapter Four). This chapter describes several types of knowledge and shows that knowledge in music therapy differs from knowledge that is presented to us through all sorts of symbols.

In Chapter Five, the first desk study that led to the idea of analogy is summarized. I made a cross-analysis of writings of music therapists and concluded that many share a proposition about why music therapy works. Their definitions were put together in the core category of analogy.

Chapter Six contains a journey into psychology and art theory. After a first draft of the core category of analogy had been made, I tried to connect the theory of analogy with psychology and art therapy. Daniel Stern's developmental psychology and semiology turned out to be bodies of knowledge that can ground analogy in psychology as well as art theory. At the same time, I continued reanalyzing and redefining the core category of analogy. In Chapter Seven, this continuous process of defining and redefining is described. Although it seems as if a final definition has been reached, this process never will come to an end.

Chapter Eight illustrates the analogy of interpersonal processes and music therapy interaction by means of two cases. The first case is the well-known case of Edward, by Paul Nordoff and Clive Robbins. The second case has been taken from my own single-case research studies. It is the case of Ingrid, the woman who locked herself in a cage.

Chapter Nine gives more examples from clinical practice to illustrate the trustworthiness of the theory of analogy. All examples were the result of single-case research studies.

Chapter Ten describes possibilities in how to research the theory of analogy by means of qualitative naturalistic research.

Finally Chapter Eleven closes with a discussion of comments on the theory of analogy that have been put forward by colleagues in the last decade.

I hope that this book inspires you to exchange ideas about the essence of music therapy. This essence must be experienced to know what it is. But we need words, too. When describing music therapy, we should be careful to use those words that are closest to the intimate music therapy experience. The theory of analogy should be a tool that helps people to experience music therapy.

Sounding the Self:
Analogy in Improvisational Music Therapy

PART I:

RESEARCH AND THEORY
IN
MUSIC THERAPY

Chapter One

MULTIPLE PERSPECTIVES ON THE DEVELOPMENT OF AN EVIDENCE-BASED MUSIC THERAPY: A PERSONAL HISTORY[1]

INTRODUCTION

For many years, I have been involved with music therapy, theory, and research. Looking back, I see several stages I went through. They show how I changed my perspective in my attempts to tighten the scientific fundamentals of music therapy. Although these stages reflect my personal development, I think they represent general perspectives through which the increase of the body of knowledge of all arts therapies (drama therapy, music therapy, art therapy, dance and movement therapy) takes place.

In this chapter, these stages will be described with examples from music therapy. I will describe the art-based perspective as well as the psycho-therapeutically based one.

I will go into the development of client-focused goals and methods, "evidence-based" rationales, qualitative and quantitative research methodologies, and, finally, the development of a general theory. At first, the various stages follow each other neatly one after the other, but toward the end, we often find the stages paralleling one another. I shall maintain a stage model for the sake of clarity, and give some examples of persons who have been involved with publications that fit into each stage. Some stages reflect historical perspectives that now seem to be outdated, whereas other stages still are very up to date.

I see a high-speed development within the immediate past that has led the profession to the threshold of scientific legitimization.

---

[1]This chapter has been presented during conferences in the Netherlands (2001), Germany (2001), and Luxembourg (2001) and has been included in conference proceedings.

THE DEVELOPMENT OF RESEARCH TOPICS IN MUSIC THERAPY

Stage One: Finding Out What Effect Music Has on the Body and the Psyche

This first foray into the profession was aimed at investigating and making an inventory of the effects that the medium of music has on people in general. One can be curious about how music is perceived, how it is processed cognitively, what feelings it elicits, how it makes subconscious experiences conscious, how it affects certain parts of the brain, and the way in which music influences neurotransmitters and vegetative reactions.

Such data from music psychology and music neurology belong to the "body of knowledge" of music therapy. Nonetheless, they do not answer the question of why music has a therapeutic effect for certain psychological disorders and handicaps. In conversations with fellow investigators, I noticed that test results had little meaning if the test did not involve clients.

The fundamental knowledge gleaned from music psychology, music neurology, general psychology and neurology, developmental psychology, psychotherapy, and psychiatry functions equally well as a theoretical touchstone to explain the effects that appear as a result of music therapy (see Stage Seven).

Some examples of research on the effects of music on the body and the psyche[2]: Hevner (1936), Reinecke (1967), Harrer (1975), Clynes (1982), Deutsch (1982), Sloboda (1985), Behne (1986), Zalanowski & Stratton (1989), Gembris (1991), Dowling (1993), Spitzer (2002), and many more.

Stage Two: Giving Music Therapy Methods a Place Within the Existing Psychotherapeutic Models

It is important to gain some insight into methods of music therapy before following the path of the investigation to diagnosis-specific effects. In order to avoid a random piling-up of methods, I decided to use a general therapeutic or psychotherapeutic classification system. The question for investigation that I deduced from this was: "How can existing methods of music therapy find a place within the existing psychotherapeutic frameworks?" These frameworks, with their assumptions about the psyche, the processes of change, and

[2]I give only some examples, not a complete overview. Years of publication have been added for historical reasons. Publications of these (well-known) authors are not included in the list of references.

interventions, served as a classification system for music therapy.

Starting with the descriptions of their work given by music therapists themselves, I classified the methods as Gestalt-therapeutic, psychoanalytic, client-centered, behavioristic, and so on. I looked for figure and background, projection and transference, empathy and unconditional positive regard, and many other concepts in the current psychotherapeutic schools of thought.

It turned out not to be so difficult to set up such a classification, even when music therapists who were seriously opposed to psychotherapy were concerned. My position was that even they who do not claim working within a psychotherapeutic frame are still influencing the psyche, and thus work psychotherapeutically. For instance, this caused me to classify the Nordoff-Robbins method as client-centered psychotherapy.

Still, this classification was not very satisfying. After a while, it became clear to me that thinking based on existing psychotherapies resulted in a set of terms not belonging to the medium of music. The concepts that were spread over music therapy (and the other arts therapies as well) covered it like a blanket. This blanket could very well suffocate such a therapy, and the validity of the classification has by no means been proven. If arts therapists label their work with concepts from psychotherapeutic schools of thought, this will not guarantee the validity of these concepts, but has more to do with what you see and what you think you see happening in your medium.

When I read publications written by music (psycho)therapists, I keep wondering if they use a theoretical framework as a legitimization toward the outside world or if this framework of terms truly fits what they are doing. Legitimization is important, but it must be done in language that outsiders can understand while it does justice to the medium. A theory must be "grounded"; that is to say, music therapists must generate concepts within the practice of the profession.

However, I did not react by embracing a purely medium-oriented approach, which seemed to me equally unsatisfactory. I was against music therapists labeling what they do with murky psychotherapeutic terms. I was just as much against music therapists going to the other extreme and assuming that the medium of music can only be described with parameters from the medium itself. The latter perspective leads to assuming that events in the medium cannot be viewed as a psychological process or--worse--that psychological processes must be named with purely musical terms. I consider metaphoric language, in which, for example, the "harmony" of the person and the "harmony" of the music are identified with each other, to be an unscientific, unpsychological, semantic approach. Metaphors can play an important role in therapy if the client experiences these metaphors. However, without the client experiencing these metaphors consciously, they cannot serve as an axiomatic explanation for the effect of music on the psyche. He who claims that music works because there is "harmony" in both music and man is not reasoning psychologically. Such "theorctical" models are very persistent in music therapy. Passionate pseudoacademics still try to explain the effect of music with the aid of notions that can be traced back to the medieval suggestion that *Musica Instrumentalis, Musica Humana,* and *Musica Mundana* are all equal.

Thus, in the course of time, I was satisfied neither with the psychotherapeutic approach nor with a purely music-oriented approach. Then it occurred to me that a "mediating" language should exist between the two, which, on the one hand, should make it possible to say clearly that what happens in the music most certainly has to do with psychology, but, on the other hand, does not alienate what is really going on in the musical processes. Thus, it should be a language that both the psychologist and the music therapist recognize. It would take a while before I could develop a theory that would make the match between music and psyche possible. Some examples:

- of attempts to categorize methods of music therapy: Strobel & Huppmann (1978), Decker-Voigt et al. (1983, 1996), Schwabe (1986), Bruscia (1987, 1989), Bruhn (2000).
- of attempts to categorize methods of music therapy within psychotherapeutic models: Schalkwijk (1984), Ruud & Mahns (1991), Smeijsters (1991/1994).

Stage Three: Tuning Music Therapy to the Client's Situation

The next step was to let go of the general effect of music (Stage One) and the general psychotherapeutic frameworks (Stage Two). My train of thought revolved around the question of how to develop diagnosis-specific methods of music therapy.

I divided the question into parts: What is the client's problem, specifically with regard to characteristic symptoms and background psychodynamics? What methodological principles, work methods, and techniques do music therapists use in their work with clients with these problems? Is it possible to deduce generally valid work methods and techniques from a comparison of approaches of a number of music therapists?

To answer these questions, I studied the quantitative and qualitative research results and case studies of a number of music therapists. I did a cross-analysis in which I compared diverse sources. In fact, I used the research technique known as triangulation in qualitative research.

Thus, my research question was no longer related to the question what psychotherapeutic framework music therapists use, but to these questions: How do they work with these problems? Is the treatment effective? What methodological conclusions can we draw? This made my approach much more critical, which was a beginning for formulating concrete criteria for effectiveness.

On the basis of the cross-analysis, I developed provisional methods for treating schizophrenia, depression, mental handicaps, autism, self-mutilation, Alzheimer's disease, anorexia, and borderline personality disorder. The methods are provisional because the material available was limited.

The question that still remained was whether it was possible to develop diagnosis-specific methods. He who looks directly through the methods for the various problem areas discovers similarities that could give the impression that music therapists do the same thing with different problems. Undoubtedly this is so up to a point. The different problems with which the clients wrestle can cause secondary problems that are not specific to the primary ones. The danger that comes with this train of thought is that music therapists may fall back on a non–diagnosis-oriented way of working.

Some examples of music therapists who developed diagnosis-specific methods: Willms (1975), Alvin (1978), Boxill (1985), Nordoff & Robbins (1983, 1986), Loos (1986), Gustorff (1990), Strobel (1990), Bruscia (1991), Goll (1993), Kapteina (1993), Robarts, Sloboda & Rogers (1995), Renz (1996), Mahns (1997), Müller & Petzold (1997), Aldridge (1996, 1999), Hibben (1999), Haffa-Schmidt, Von Moreau & Wölfl (1999), Schumacher (1994, 1999), Smeijsters (1995, 1996, 1997, 1999), Wigram et al. (1993, 1995, 1999), and many more.

Stage Four: Criteria for Developing an Evidence-Based Indication

The criteria that I set up for music therapy became, as already said, gradually more concrete. National discussions, among other things, convinced me of the principle that it is better to claim less that can be proved than to claim much that cannot be proved. Picture this point of view before the background in which all therapies in the mental health care services in the Netherlands critically were being assessed. The demand to concentrate on the things one does well became louder and louder. The suggestion that music therapy could do everything for everybody simply had no credibility. Music therapy had gradually become adult, and, on that account, could no longer afford escaping scientific criteria. Some while before this, I had already abandoned the idea that music therapy had a right to exist as long as it looked like psychotherapy and could be described with psychotherapeutic terminology (see Stage Two).

A model for determining an indication gradually crystallized in my mind. Determining an "indication" means answering the question of whether a specific therapeutic method is appropriate for the client's specific problem. I developed a number of subquestions that need to be answered positively if one claims that music therapy is the right therapy in the right place and the right time.[3] These subquestions are as follows:

1) What is the client's problem?
2) What goals and methods are suitable for the client's problem? Does music therapy fit in with these goals?
3) Does music therapy help to reach these goals? What effects does music therapy have?
4) Is there a credible theoretical explanation for the effects of music therapy that is corroborated by theoretical models of psychology and psychotherapy?
5) What conditions must be met to make music therapy a success for this client?

If all five of these criteria have been fulfilled, you might claim that music therapy indeed is the appropriate therapy for the client's problem. I am sure that some of my colleagues think this list of questions is too strict. So little research has been done that the result could be negative even if it were clinically evident that music therapy has had a positive effect.

The questions are not intended to take away the right of existence of arts therapies, but to strengthen that right. The questions are a task for the future. And, should it be that there is enough clinical evidence that arts therapies are effective, then it is important to collect and systematize this evidence in a scientific manner. Question 3 makes an indication "evidence-based" because it asks for effects that are the result of quantitative, qualitative, and/or comparative research.

Examples of work that addresses the questions for indication include Smeijsters (1995/1999b, 2000/2003). The next chapter will discuss indications in more detail.

Stage Five: Categorizing the Goals

Question 2 of the indication model led to a separate stage in which I dealt with the question of whether it is possible to categorize the goals that music therapists set for themselves. I felt that this question is important because it

[3]In fact, these criteria can be applied to all (arts) therapies.

makes the music therapist's work more transparent for others. It is true that there are many connecting links between the activities of the various music therapists, but there are also differing elements. The goals one tries to achieve form such an element.

I used Wolberg's (1977) and Wheeler's (1987) classification in the supportive, re-educative and reconstructive categories, and added the palliative category and the developmental category for the handicapped. Each category consists of goals that are closely related. There are several other classifications in circulation, such as the classification of De Jonghe et al. (1987/1988), which in the Netherlands has been used for testing so-called treatment products for arts therapies. The classifications seem to correlate well, apart from the difference in terminology.

The classification makes it possible to map out the goals--which are connected to methods, activities, and techniques--of the music therapist. Some music therapists work mainly with one particular category of goals, others alternate between categories, and still others use categories in parallel. The squabbling of music therapists among themselves and other professionals about who is really entitled to call himself a music therapist, and who is not, is now largely in the past, thanks to the classification method. Music therapy is a concept that bridges various working methods.

Examples of classifications of goals: Schwabe (1986), Wheeler (1983, 1987), Schalkwijk (1988), Bruscia (1989/1998), Smeijsters (2000/2003), Drieschner & Pioch (2000).

Stage Six: Analyzing Suitable Research Methods for Music Therapy

This question, which I have continually asked myself in my many years of research, consists of two parts:

1) What research methods are suitable for determining effects?
2) What research methods are suitable for developing a "grounded theory" for music therapy?

To answer these questions, I evaluated differing types of quantitative research, and I mapped out their possibilities and impossibilities for music therapy. I also studied, systematized, and evaluated a large number of qualitative research methods. The qualitative research methods, such as phenomenology, grounded theory, naturalistic inquiry, and hermeneutics, are rapidly gaining international attention in music therapy.

In the '90s, a qualitative research group was formed in the world of music therapy that consists mainly of researchers who completely reject quantitative research. They do not do this because of unfamiliarity with quantitative methodology; on the contrary, they base this on the experience that this methodology cannot satisfactorily describe what happens in music therapy.

I myself took an intermediate position in this discussion. I think that it is not sensible to throw the quantitative research overboard. There is no objection to measuring in a quantitative way the effects of music therapy, no matter how limited these measurements may be. Quantitative research has its own questions and has its own outcome, which contribute to the legitimization of the therapy. If it is not possible to prove the effects in a quantitative way somehow, then the therapy has no right to exist. One cannot maintain that a therapy is effective if it is never statistically significant in a quantitative investigation. I consider quantitative research a coarse sieve: A lot falls through the holes, but if you are to legitimize what you are doing, then at least something must be left in the sieve.

However, this does not mean that the quantitative paradigm does not receive a lot of criticism. Efficacy research is reductionistic with respect to the client, the therapist, and the method, and therefore what it can detect strongly has weak validity. The efficacy design does not mirror regular treatment due to standardization.

Especially, the reductionism is severely criticized by music therapists because it causes the essence of music therapy to disappear behind standardization and simple models of variables. By the "essence" of the therapy, I mean the complex, multilayered activities and experiences of the client and the music therapist.

The qualitative paradigm can have flaws too, as when, for instance, the accent on "subjectivity" and "experience" leads to the assumption that only the music therapist knows exactly what is happening, because he is the one who during therapy experiences the empathetic countertransference. This question can be solved with the hypothesis that therapy is indeed about the subjective experiences of the music therapist and the client, but this, however, does not imply that there are no methodological criteria with which to register and analyze these experiences.

The perspective of qualitative research shed a new light on the psychotherapeutic framework. Because I was using qualitative methods such as phenomenology, naturalistic inquiry, and grounded theory, I put off forming a theory as long as possible--until the empirical data pushed me in the direction of certain ideas that I could no longer avoid. So it could happen that concepts from client-centered psychotherapy popped up in one stage of music therapy treatment, and concepts from object-relation therapy popped up in another stage. I made it a principle never to start an investigation with a fixed framework of concepts. Concepts were generated from the research material in the memos. As we see in the next section, the qualitative paradigm has been used also when developing the general theory of music therapy that forms the main part of this book.

Examples on research methodology: Tüpker (1990), Wheeler (1995), Aldridge (1996), Langenberg (1996), Bolay, Boller, Czogalik & Kächele (1997), Smeijsters (1996, 1997), Ansdell & Pavlicevic (2001), Kächele et al. (1989–2001). See also these examples from other therapies: drama, Grainger (1999); art, McNiff (1998); dance and movement, Higgins (1993).

Stage Seven: Developing a Theoretical Model of Explanation

Once I had mapped out the research methodologies, the question of which theoretical model could explain the effects of music therapy became important. On the basis of my earlier searches in which I compared empirical material with theoretical frameworks, I concluded that the usual psychotherapeutic trains of thought and the art therapeutic theories either explain only a part of the psychological processes of music therapy or lean too heavily on the process of artistic creation, which only roughly corresponds to the therapeutic process. I went looking for a theory that could make a direct connection between what happens in the music activity and in the client's psyche.

Before the theory of analogy appeared on the horizon, which will be worked out in Part II of this book, I collected many examples of therapeutic processes in the music from my own research and that of others. It was evident from these examples that what occurred in the music activity correlated closely with the way the client behaved and what he experienced in general. I particularly valued the experience of the clients themselves that such a correlation exists, and I did this from the viewpoint of the research technique of "member checking." Nonetheless, I realized that member checking is not possible for every target group, and, therefore, validation is difficult.

A theory does not just fall out of a clear blue sky. In the music therapy literature, I looked for explanations of the way music therapy works given by music therapists themselves. The explanations I was looking for were not those borrowed from grand theories, but less abstract answers to the question of why music therapy works.

I compared these explanations with one another and discovered that music therapists who work with the most divergent theoretical schools of thought have similar basic explanations for the way music therapy works. I call this basal--still rudimentary--theory, "the theory of analogy." This theory is a "grounded theory" because it has a two-part foundation in practice. On the one hand, it is founded on concrete processes that take place in music activities during music therapy. On the other hand, it is founded on music therapist's statements about these processes.

In the first place, an analogy describes the similarity between the psychological characteristics of the client and the way the client expresses himself in the music. In the second place, it describes the similarity between the change in the music and the psychological change in the client.

The advantage of this theoretical model is that it leaves room for both the variation among individual clients and the variation among different methodological approaches. "The" analogy does not exist. Each of the client's problems has its own analogous processes in the music. Each client, each therapist, and each method fits in this model. In this theory, it is very important that a direct connection can be made between what happens visibly and audibly in the music and what happens in the psyche.

At first, I was surprised that I could develop a common theory for music therapists working with diverse theoretical frameworks. I was surprised again when I realized that Daniel Stern's developmental psychology gives the theory of analogy a general psychological foundation.

Stern (1985) explains the early interaction between child and caregiver by analogy. One can speak of an analogy because there is a similarity between the basal psychological processes of the child and the way in which these processes are expressed in different modalities such as movement, sound, and image. If the "vitality affects" of the psyche, the basal processes that take place within the psyche, are determined by parameters such as form, intensity, movement, number, and rhythm, the door to music (and other arts therapies) is wide open. When I realized this, many pieces of the music therapy puzzle fell into place. It is interesting that no "foreign" theory is brought into this therapy except for psychology, which in itself uses musical parameters, as a foundation.

In the past I have often had interesting discussions with students about the need for theory. The main question was how important it is to make a theory trustworthy. Students with a practical style of learning often have the tendency to reason that what is important is that it works, and of course this is what the music therapist aims for. If, however, this bent toward practicality leads to producing the most obscure and fuzzy theories in order to explain the effect, then the door to scientific legitimization remains closed. Theories of music therapy (and all arts therapies) must correlate with the results of other theories about how and why people change.

Examples of theories that have been developed to explain the effects of music therapy: Benenzon (1983), Priestley (1983), Nordoff & Robbins (1986), Kenny (1989), Knill (1987, 1990), Hegi (1986, 1998), Schwabe (1986), Strobel (1990), Frohne-Hagemann (1990), Lecourt (1994), Mastnak (1994), Langenberg (1995), Tüpker & Weymann (1988, 1990, 1996), Niedecken (1996), Pavlicevic (1997), Smeijsters (1999, 2000/2003), and many more.

Stage Eight: A Framework Covering All Arts Therapies

Although this book is about music therapy, I will shortly go into my work for the arts therapies, which also is of interest to music therapists. I have finally integrated and applied all the preceding steps to the arts therapies (drama therapy, music therapy, art therapy, and dance and movement therapy).

Framework terms that I have used in this are the CT molecule, the clinical reasoning process, the psychology of the medium, and analogy.

By "CT molecule," I mean a coherent whole of components with which arts therapists have to deal: the psychological development and neuropsychology of the human being; psychological problems that can occur during a lifetime; relevant treatment goals; the question of whether art therapy is indicated to reach treatment goals; the core therapeutic processes of thc arts therapies; inherent therapeutic possibilities of the specific media (drama, music, art, dance and movement); methods, activities, and techniques of the arts therapies; the organizational context in which arts therapists work; arts therapies as a profession; and, finally, researching the arts therapies. The CT molecule can serve as a framework for education and research, because each component can be a focus of education and research.

The CT molecule is in fact a detailed elaboration of the three segments as they are described in the profile of the profession of the Dutch Association for Creative Therapy and the profile for national training and higher vocational education:

> Segment One: Working with the client
> Segment Two: Working within an organization
> Segment Three: The development of the profession and the body of knowledge

The "clinical reasoning process" refers to the cohesion of the components of the CT molecule. It is the process that takes place in the mind of the "reflective practitioner" (Argyris & Schön, 1978), which moves step by step from one component to the next by means of argumentation. In this way, it determines what he brings about by whom, and how and why he does it. The clinical reasoning process has a lot in common with the reasoning process of the (qualitative) researcher.

The "psychology of the medium" refers to the description and analysis of the client's process in the medium in a way that makes transparent the client's psychological process. The psychology of the medium needs a language that is an intermediate between medium language and psychological language so that it will be possible that in the same time arts therapists as well as psychotherapists can understand the client's therapeutic process.

For me, the theory of analogy became the connecting theoretical instrument in the arts therapies. I analyzed the effects of the various arts therapies, and I looked for theoretical explanations that fit these effects best. At the beginning, I considered this as a daring undertaking of which the outcome was totally uncertain. Would the theory of analogy also be valid for other arts therapies? Finally, I found enough evidence that makes it likely that the concept of analogy is valid for all arts therapies. However, the last word about this has not been spoken. Much supplementary research is needed. The central questions are: Which medium processes can change the behavior and experience of the client in the medium in such a way that the client's condition is improved? Can this be explained by means of analogy? For some years now, I have had students of all arts therapies carry out a qualitative investigation of analogies in their final year of training (see Chapter Ten). I would like to see the theory of analogy tested in everyday practice in various target groups by independent practitioners.

Source: Smeijsters, (2000/2003). Other examples of theories covering all arts therapies: Wils (1973), Knill (1979, 1992), Petzold (1988), Smitskamp and Te Velde (1988), Aldridge, Brandt & Wohler (1990).

THE AGENDA FOR THE FUTURE: PEER DEBRIEFING

My approach changed in the course of the years. Instead of undertaking an individual journey of discovery, I joined forces with others. I had applied the qualitative research technique of "peer debriefing" to my own empirical research by submitting my results and conclusions to independent experts. Now I launched the technique into a wider context.

I welcomed contact with the practitioners during these years with the purpose of integrating the practical knowledge of the various arts therapists and testing the ideas I myself developed in practice. The feeling that I was a pioneer, exploring unknown territory on his own and hoping to discover beautiful landscapes, gave way to the notice that the arts therapies had to rise above the pioneer stage.

After the stage in which fervent individuals develop their methods and theories on their own, there must follow a stage in which the development of methods and theories no longer depends on single individuals. The development of the body of knowledge should be anchored in a professional and scientific community that is consensus-based.

I predict that the profession's future depends on the degree(s) of research activity coordination and systematic communication achieved by researchers.

Chapter Two

CRITERIA FOR INDICATIONS IN MUSIC THERAPY

INTRODUCTION

In the Netherlands, the health care system has become more "evidence based." The arts therapists working in clinical institutions are urged to defend the arts therapies and give a straight answer on questions such as, "Why should there be arts therapies for this particular client or client group?"

If you want to answer this question, you need criteria that can assure you that the question has been answered adequately. Thus, these criteria are very important in the discussion of how important music therapy (and the other arts therapies) can be in health care. For that reason, one of the stages in my own scientific development focused on the development of criteria for indications.

Indication criteria refer to reasons *why* arts therapies can be applied there. Indication criteria are not the areas of disturbances or handicaps where arts therapies can be applied. Criteria guide the act of reasoning that should be carried out to judge the application of arts therapies. This act of reasoning should be guided by questions that need to be answered and that in the end decide whether there are enough reasons to conclude that arts therapies should be applied in a specific area.

In this chapter, I will describe which steps have been undertaken to define a set of criteria for indications. Although these criteria have been developed within a music therapy project, in my opinion the results are of relevance for all arts therapies. Therefore, in the following text I will generalize to all arts therapies wherever this is possible, and refer to the music therapy project as an example.

I will describe the research that has been undertaken to test the criteria, give some examples of indications, and, finally, discuss traps when answering the question of whether arts therapies are indicated.

RESEARCH

Method

ON THE NATIONAL LEVEL. Analyzing case studies of Dutch music therapists, investigating how--up until 1990--they made use of indications, was the first step. In 1991, I developed a set of criteria for indications that was used during a postgraduate course for music therapists from different working areas in the Netherlands.

ON THE INTERNATIONAL LEVEL. This set of criteria was also discussed during a Round Table Meeting on indications during the 3rd European Music Therapy Congress in Aalborg (1995). As a follow-up, a second draft of criteria was then sent out to several members of the Aalborg Round Table Group, together with a questionnaire (Van den Berk, 1996). Those members were representatives from different countries: the Netherlands (Van Nieuwenhuijzen), United Kingdom (Odell-Miller), Argentina (Schapira), and Denmark (Steen Moeller).

I made an analysis of the answers to questions in the questionnaire that were connected to indications. During a Round Table Meeting at the 8th World Congress of Music Therapy in Hamburg (1996), the second draft of criteria and the results from the questionnaire were discussed with representatives from countries all over the world.

Results: On the National Level

QUALITATIVE ANALYSIS. From my own qualitative analysis of music therapy case studies, several conclusions could be drawn, such as:

- Music therapists, when arguing why music therapy should be used, often make nonspecific statements not telling why they are recommending music therapy
- When specific effects of music therapy are mentioned, it often is not clear why these effects should be used with this particular disturbance or handicap
- When specific effects of music are mentioned, most of the time there is no sound theoretical explanation or scientific evidence that makes trustworthy the proposed effect
- Often, music therapy is offered because the client loves music

Rebergen (1992, 1993) did a comparative research on all arts therapies, and asked himself, "What is the best type of art therapy for a client with a borderline disturbance?" To find the answer, he made a qualitative analysis of writings of arts therapists and other professionals. His findings show that arts therapists—during the early '90s—described their goals so broadly that it would seem as if every client could benefit from arts therapies.

Arts therapists in this study, in my opinion, focus on secondary health problems of the client and not on primary therapeutic needs (see Bruscia, 1989/1998). Goals such as "creativity," "actualization," "growth," "experiment," and "play" are so broad that they can be used with almost everybody, at any time, in any place. However, these goals cannot prove the primary therapeutic significance of the arts therapies for the borderline client. For instance, there is a lack of evidence that "stimulating the client's creativity" indeed alleviates his feeling of being abandoned, his emotional instability, his weak identity, and so on.

From the results of Rebergen, it becomes clear that the arts therapists he researched were unable to define when and why their particular type of therapy is indicated for the client's problems, and when it is not (contraindication).

The results of another study show that it is difficult to describe the differences and commonalities of arts therapies. Gieles, De Jager, and Van Laarhoven (1997) asked arts therapists to describe their assessment foci and their treatment goals. From their material I made a cross-analysis, comparing assessment foci and goals from different arts therapists. The results of this analysis show:

- Many overlaps in assessment foci
- Overlaps in treatment goals
- That several times arts therapies during assessment have foci that are not transferred into treatment goals
- That in some cases it was proposed that assessment foci and treatment goals belong to specific types of arts therapies

Because the Gieles et al. study was a survey of opinions, checking the propositions made by individual arts therapies, several questions should be raised:

- Do the overlaps in assessment foci make arts therapies equally effective in assessment?
- Do the overlaps in treatment goals make arts therapies equally effective in treatment?
- Do some assessment foci and treatment goals belong to specific types of arts therapies as proposed?

These conclusions and questions brought me to the idea that criteria for indications are needed, by which in a sound way it can be concluded why, when, and to whom arts therapies should be offered.

THE PROPOSED CRITERIA FOR INDICATIONS. To make sure that music therapy as a treatment is indicated, whether it is the "right therapy for the right person," a music therapist should ask himself the following questions.

What is the client's problem? If you claim that music therapy helps the client, you first have to go into the client's problem. If you do not research the client's problem, you will be unable afterward to conclude whether music therapy helped the client to overcome his problem.

What goals and methods are suitable for the client's problem? Does music therapy fit in with these goals? If you know the client's problem, you should ask yourself what goals should be reached, and if there are methods, activities, and techniques in music therapy by which these goals can be reached. Part of this question is to decide which treatment modality is needed and whether music therapy meets the criteria of this treatment modality. The choice of treatment modality depends on the description of the disturbance or handicap (see first question) and on general therapeutic principles. Examples of treatment modalities for music therapy are developmental music therapy, rehabilitative music therapy, supportive music therapy, palliative music therapy, re-educative music therapy and reconstructive music therapy (adopted and adjusted from Wheeler, 1983 and 1987, Bruscia 1989; see also Schalkwijk 1994). Research from other therapeutic fields shows that for a disturbance or handicap, a specific treatment modality often is most appropriate. Thus the music therapist should ask himself:

a) Whether he is choosing the most appropriate treatment modality and
b) Whether music methods, activities, and techniques of music therapy fit into this treatment modality

Does music therapy help to reach these goals? What effects does music therapy have? If you think that music therapy has methods, activities, and techniques to help the client reach the goals, then you should consider whether there is some clinical and/or research evidence that these goals indeed have been reached by means of music therapy elsewhere. To answer this question, the music therapist should investigate case studies and research findings to find data that show that music therapy, when using the appropriate treatment modality (see second question) with the disturbance or handicap (see first question), indeed has significant effects. These data can also be found in treatment protocols of one's own clinical experiences. Another way to look at this question is arguing that music therapy is indicated because it has specific characteristics that make it more appropriate than other therapies. This can be done by: a) using the results of discriminative research, or b) developing arguments about differences between music therapy and other types of therapies.

Is there a credible theoretical explanation for the effects of music therapy that is corroborated by theoretical models of psychology and psychotherapy? This criterion tells you that when criteria 1-2-3 have bean met, you need a theoretical framework that explains why music therapy helps the client to overcome his problem. Music therapists should develop a theory that can explain the particular effects of music therapy. This theory needs to be linked to other theoretical models, which can be inferred, from neurology, psychiatry, psychology, and so on. For example, when in music therapy the use of songs in working with clients who suffer from expressive aphasia leads to a more fluent language (an effect which is subsumed under question three), one can use the theory about the brain hemispheres to explain this effect.

What conditions must be met to make music therapy a success for this client? Finally, if all previous criteria have been met, you should consider whether your particular client has enough resources to join music therapy. For instance, is your client able to participate in activities? Is he affiliated to music?

Basic to the criteria of indication is the idea that each time a music therapist thinks that music therapy should be offered, he needs to ask himself, "What reason is there that music therapy should be used?" The criteria are meant to make this question easier to be answered. In my opinion, we need to take the criteria for indications very seriously if we want to offer the best to our clients. The next section gives some examples of how the criteria can be used.

Results: On the International Level

ANALYSIS OF THE QUESTIONNAIRE ON CRITERIA FOR INDICATIONS. The analysis of the questionnaire shows that music therapists are used to answering questions of indication by naming areas of work (for example: depression) where in their opinion music therapy can be used. In their written comments on indication, they do not reflect treatment modalities or research effects. Theoretical considerations (rationales) often are missing or lack a sound theoretical background.

For music therapists, it seems to be unclear what is meant by criteria for indications. Criteria for indications force you to find arguments WHY music therapy should be used with a client. When a music therapist states, "Music therapy is indicated for depression," then this sentence should be the final conclusion of a process of reasoning. He should be able to say, "Music therapy is indicated for depression *because ...*"

The results from the questionnaire showed also that there is some misunderstanding about referral, assessment, and indication. In a referral, a colleague of another profession assigns the client to music therapy. This referral should include a rationale for why the client has been referred to music therapy. The music therapist, by means of an assessment, makes a supplementary diagnosis of the client, researches the rationale for why the client has been referred, and gives a final rationale as to why music therapy is appropriate.

The questionnaire showed further that music therapists, when mentioning areas of work, make use of different category systems. One system focuses on categories of disturbances and handicaps (neurosis, psychosis, manic depression, psychotrauma, eating problems, sexual abuse, dementia, HIV, the physically handicapped, the mentally handicapped, and so on), whereas another category focuses on psychological functions (emotion, cognition, perception, social behavior, self-esteem, language, and so on).

Disturbed functions may be symptoms of disturbances and handicaps. Nevertheless, the question remains as to whether we should concentrate on, for instance, emotional aspects in general, or whether we should focus on emotional aspects of, for example, depression in particular. In other words, the argument that music therapy is indicated in the field of emotion is not the adequate rationale when one wants to claim that music therapy is an appropriate therapy for depression.

The Criteria for Indications in Practice

The set of criteria has been used in educational and clinical settings in the Netherlands, in Germany, and other European countries (with psychiatric populations, the mentally handicapped, and autistic clients). During a symposium in the fall of 1997, several music therapists working in Germany presented papers that showed how the criteria of indications could be used in practice. From their clinical experience, Krantz (1997) and Krantz and Van der Poel (1997) defined a sixth criterion: the organizational setting in which the music therapist works. They point out that the music therapist's indication is influenced and even limited by the treatment philosophy (goals, duration, therapeutic modality, and therapeutic model) that is leading within the clinic. They also described that in clinical practice the criteria of indications do not follow a linear course from criterion one to five or six, but go through different sequences (for instance, 6-3-4-5-1-4-2). In their opinion, criterion six (the organizational context) is where it all starts. Hafkamp (1997) introduced the indication criteria in her work with the developmentally handicapped. She brought forward that because of clinical workload and time limits, it is not possible to go through all criteria with each client.

Nygaard Pedersen (1999) has been following the indication criteria in her work with schizophrenic and psychotic clients strictly. When fulfilling the third criterion, she made a cross-analysis of her own case material that makes clear that each music therapist, without complex research designs, can answer this criterion by means of clinical experience. When fulfilling the fourth criterion, she made a link to theories on schizophrenia developed by outstanding psychiatrists and psychologists, thus making use of theoretical triangulation. All these examples show how reflective practitioners can ground a systematically theoretical reflection in clinical practice.

In the end, it seems that the criteria for indications are needed and useful to guide the work of the music therapist, if they are adjusted to practice. The criteria should be used flexibly, which means that some questions can be answered more in general; some other questions need to be answered for each particular client. Also, the sequence should be different from context to context. As with most guidelines, they should help the therapist make his work stronger, and not lock his therapeutic behavior in a cage.

To me, it is essential that the music therapist as a reflective practitioner continuously should go through a process of clinical reasoning in which all criteria are met. Each treatment should continuously be questioned as to whether it is the appropriate treatment for the needs of this client and whether the goals are reached, and so on. As Krantz points out, in practice often it works the other way around: The music therapist is forced to describe his method, and then it is asked, "Who is the right client for music therapy?" This *should* be: "Which type of music therapy can the client benefit from?" Only the latter question leads to adjusting over and over again the music therapy method to the needs of our clients, and thus can give the clients what they came for.

EXAMPLES OF INDICATIONS

In Table 2.1, I will give an example of how the criteria for indication can be met in the case of music therapy aimed at improving the social contact of clients with schizophrenia. Please remember that fulfilling the criteria gives you only a general idea of whether music therapy is indicated. The information in this and the forthcoming tables should be used carefully. These tables are not manuals, because the treatment always should be attuned to the individual characteristics and needs of the client. This table can only give some sort of a direction for treatment.

Table 2.1

Indications for Schizophrenia—
Especially Improving Social Contact

Disturbance
- Chronic schizophrenia, residual type

Negative Symptoms
- Flattening of affect, poverty of thinking and speech, apathy (DSM-IV), social withdrawal, lack of initiative (Andreasen, 1982)

Treatment Goal
- The treatment of social withdrawal

General Treatment
- The psychiatric rehabilitation treatment modality for chronic patients focuses on the reduction of negative symptoms, especially the improvement of social interaction (Anthony & Liberman, 1986; Coursey, 1989; Liberman, DeRisi, & Mueser, 1989; Wasylenki, 1992).

Music Therapy Treatment
- Rehabilitative music therapy focuses on becoming aware of another person, increases adjustment, and improves cooperation. It does not aim at the exploration of feelings or the increase of insight (Smeijsters, 2000/2003). See also the holding and reorganizing treatment modality developed by Nygaard Pedersen (1999), for work with schizophrenic clients, with the aims of breaking the isolation and communicating.

Effects of Music Therapy as a Result of Research or Clinical Practice
- In an experimental study in practice by Pfeiffer, Wunderlich, Bender, Elz, and Horn (1987), a mix of musical improvisation and talking with schizophrenic clients resulted in significant improvement in clients' self-reports concerning their social ability.
- Nine weekly sessions of active individual music therapy improved the musical interaction between the chronic schizophrenic client and the music therapist significantly when compared with a matched control group (Pavlicevic, Trevarthen, & Duncan, 1994). Parallel to this there was a significant drop on the *Brief Psychiatric Rating Scale*, and little change in the *Scale for the Assessment of Negative Symptoms*.
- Research by Perilli (1994) shows an improvement of negative symptoms on the *Nurses' Observation Scale for Inpatient Evaluation* as a result of music therapy.
- Research by Tang, Yao & Zheng (1994) shows that receptive music therapy and singing popular songs significantly diminished the clients' negative symptoms, and increased their level of interest in external events

as measured by the *Scale for Assessment for Negative Symptoms* and the *World Health Organization's Disability Assessment Scale.*

- Individual music therapy and music therapy in groups, combined with medication, decreases negative symptoms, measured by PSE, SANS, BPRS, SDSI, statistically significant, compared to a control group with medication only. The effects are stable (Yang et al, 1998).
- A case study by Jensen (1999) gives evidence that a schizophrenic client is able to move away from the usual phrases and patterns, to respond to the music therapist's rhythm, and to play together with the music therapist.
- Receptive and active music therapy with the aim to express feelings and social interaction results in a decrease of anxiety and compulsive behaviors and an increase of social sensitivity (De l'Etoile, 2002).
- Music listening, singing in a choir and improvisation show a statistical significant improvement of negative symptoms, measured by PANSS, OLS, and REHAB, of the treatment group compared to the control group. When treatment stops the effects diminish (Hayashi et al, 2002).
- Individual music therapy with improvisation shows no statistical significant improvement of negative symptoms, measured by MUERB and MUSIKOS. However, qualitative data show that negative symptoms improve. There is no improvement outside music therapy (Buchert, 2003).
- Song composition as reinforcement for social behaviour decreases aggressive behaviour (Silverman 2003).

Effects of Other Treatment Modalities as a Result of Research or Clinical Practice

- Insight-oriented psychotherapy and group psychotherapy are of limited use (Gunderson et al., 1984; Van den Bosch, 1994).

The Theory and/or Hypotheses That Might Explain the Effect

- Because of cognitive impairment, schizophrenic patients have difficulties with verbal interaction. During verbal interaction, it is not the semantic meaning of words that is primarily important, but the musical characteristics of the process of interaction. Thus, meaning is less important than the sound parameters in which words are expressed: pitch, melody, tempo, rhythm, dynamics, and timbre (Benedetti, 1991; Strobel, 1990). These sound parameters are equal to emotional signals.
- In music therapy, not the verbal but the musical interaction is the primary focus. Therefore, music therapy comes close to the experience of the schizophrenic client. In music therapy, the schizophrenic client can explore the emotional-musical aspect of interaction. By this, the client is able to understand the partner, to adjust to him, and to be part of the interaction.
- In music therapy, the music therapist, by means of an ultrasensitive listening attitude that is part of a holding and reorganizing treatment

modality, listens to the client's emotional signals and enables the client to change his emotional-musical interaction (Nygaard Pedersen, 1999).
- Research about environmental factors shows how important it is that schizophrenic clients can control the emotional aspects of interaction. Research on "expressed emotion" shows that an agitated emotional environment, which is expressed in nonverbal negative emotional sounds during interaction, means a high risk of decompensation for the schizophrenic client (Leff & Vaughn, 1985)

Resources Needed by the Client
- Sufficient affinity with music
- Motivation to be enrolled in music therapy
- Some awareness of his environment
- A high enough activity level to be treated in active music therapy
- The cognitive ability to make a transfer from musical to nonmusical behavior

Table 2.2 gives an example of autism worked out during a postgraduate course.

Table 2.2

Indications for Autism—
Especially Decreasing Stereotyped Behavior[4]

Handicap
- Autism

Characteristics
- Specific: disorders related to cognition, social interaction [eye contact, facial expression, body posture, gestures, relationships with peers, sharing pleasure and play, emotional reciprocity (DSM-IV)], and communication [acquisition or variability in language, conversation, symbolic play (DSM-IV)] (Kraijer, 1991).
- Semispecific (problems that will be found often with autism, but can be found with other disorders, too): rigid, stereotyped, obsessive, overstructured, and ritualistic behaviors (Kraijer, 1991).
- Nonspecific (problems that are not typical for autism, but sometimes can be found with autism, too): hyperactive, destructive, and aggressive behaviors (Kraijer, 1991).

---

[4]This table has been developed in cooperation with Wilma Vroegop-Speelman.

Treatment Goal

- The treatment of rigid, stereotyped, obsessive, overstructured, and ritualistic behaviors

General Treatment

- Reinforcing structure by means of stimulus reduction (reducing the number of stimuli), stimulus selection (selecting just one stimulus for attention), stimulus reinforcement (giving attention to just one stimulus), stimulus regulation (working in a fixed time sequence), and stimulus extension (offering new stimuli within well-known structured stimuli) (Kraijer, 1991; Verhey & Van Loon, 1993).

Music Therapy Treatment

- Developmental music therapy aims at growth and progress in behavioral areas of functioning by means of structured play forms.

Effects of Music Therapy as a Result of Research or Clinical Practice

- Nordoff and Robbins (1977), Bryan (1982), and Weber (1991) report that it is possible to change the child's obsessive behavior by incorporating the child in the cadence of a piece of music.
- Alvin and Warwick (1991) report that it is possible to change the child's stereotyped tempo when the music therapist uses a tempo that is a little bit faster that the child's original tempo.
- Music therapists such as Weber (1991, 1996) and Lecourt (1991) report progress in stereotyped behavior when using a balance between "iso" and "provocation," "confrontation," or "alternation."
- Schulz (1987) and Lecourt report positive results when using syncopations.
- Schumacher (1994) and Weber (1996) report that pauses stimulate the child to stop stereotyped behaviors and take initiatives.
- Schumacher (1999) shows how by means of affect attunement and intermodal reactions of the music therapist a dialogue and a turn-taking of imitating and taking initiatives develops.
- Di Franco (1999) shows how focusing on the body and its expression through the voice diminishes rigidity.
- Case studies of Berger (2002), who does not focus on stereotyped behaviour directly, show that active music therapy stimulates imitation, initiative, spontaneity, creativity and variability. These are psychological phenomena that can counteract rigidity.
- Brownell (2002) shows that stories with behavioural guidelines that are sung decrease disruptive behaviours at school.

The Theory and/or Hypotheses That Might Explain the Effect

- The autistic child has deficits in the ability to structure information. Because unstructured information is a threat, the child needs redundancy. Stereotyped behavior acts as a defense that excludes unstructured informa-

tion (Rutter & Schopler, 1987; Van Engeland, 1992).
- Music can be redundant internally when it consists of a low level of information; it can be also externally redundant by means of repetition.
- The music therapist can offer one instrument (stimulus selection) play and repeat redundant music (stimulus reduction), and by this open the child to his environment, and then use a stimulus regulation technique (introducing new sounds that are embedded between well-known form parts), a stimulus reinforcing technique (attracting attention to one parameter), and a stimulus extension technique by means of the sequenced or synchronized conservation and variation principle (repeating the same music with some variations in one parameter over time or matching the child's musical behavior almost completely, but synchronously introducing variations in one parameter) (Smeijsters, 1995/1999b).

Resources Needed by the Client
- The client must be able to stay in the room.

In Table 2.3, I developed an instruction model for students in the bachelor's degree course who by means of a case from clinical practice are trained to develop an indication.

In this example, the evidence on music therapy effects that could be found in literature is limited. Nevertheless, the example shows how by means of a systematic analysis a convincing indication for music therapy can be developed.

Table 2.3

Indications for a Child With an Internalized Behavior Problem, Anxiety Modus

Diagnosis
- Internalized behavior problem, anxiety modus (Delfos, 2000)

Symptoms
- School phobia (vomiting, panic attacks, and breathing problems at school), avoiding contact, being anxious, lacking assertiveness, feeling threatened, having low self-esteem (adjusted from Petersen, 1998)

Psychodynamics
- Strong attachment to mother, vehement reaction when mother leaves, helpless when left on own, relationship problems with others

General Treatment
- Goal: increasing interaction with another (strange) person

- Modality: re-educative, with the focus on decreasing anxiety, strengthening frustration tolerance, increasing interpersonal abilities, increasing assertiveness, strengthening self-esteem
- Methods: behavior therapy (systematic desensitization), competency training (enlarging already existing competencies), therapy of phasing (enhancing trust, introducing nearness, exploring together, interaction) (Thoomes-Vreugdenhil, 2000)

Music Therapy Treatment

- Modality: re-educative music therapy with goals to strengthen frustration tolerance (acceptance of a stranger), increase interpersonal abilities (going into interaction), and express hidden feelings
- Method: analytically oriented music therapy (object relations theory; transference)
- Activities: the music therapist demonstrates musical instruments; the child plays; the music therapist acts as a listener; the music therapist supplements the child's play on instruments (Petersen, 1998).

Effects of Music Therapy as a Result of Research or Clinical Practice

- A case study shows that music therapy is able to help the child to overcome his anxiety to play loudly and freely, develop an interaction between the child and the "strange" music therapist, and attend school again when feelings of sorrow and anger have been expressed during music therapy (Petersen, 1998).

Effects of Other Treatment Modalities as a Result of Research or Clinical Practice

- Behavior therapy shows good effects in the treatment of anxiety (Emmelkamp, 1995).

The Theory and/or Hypotheses That Might Explain the Effect

- Music therapy makes it possible to express experiences from a very early stage of life that are difficult to put into words
- In the musical improvisation, the child feels in the here-and-now his problems of anxiety, low frustration tolerance, lack of interpersonal abilities, lack of assertiveness, and low self-esteem
- Music therapy makes it possible that the child goes into insecure territory, finds a secure place for herself, loosens his need for control, expresses hidden feelings, and loosens his anxiety in interacting
- Because of the fact that the music therapist gradually becomes a partner in the child's musical play, but also stays in his role of "stranger," the child--in a situation of transference--can loosen the strong attachment to his mother.

Resources Needed by the Client

- The mother or the person to whom the child is strongly attached should be able to bring the child to therapy and stay in the waiting room.

DISCUSSION

In this final part, I want to focus on several issues one should consider when searching for reasons why arts therapies are indicated.

The Danger of Essentialism and Holism

Van der Klis (1997) mentions two traps when answering the question as to why arts therapies may be indicated: essentialistic and holistic reasoning. Arts therapists using *essentialistic* reasoning claim that arts therapies are indicated because the human being in essence is a mover, a dancer, a music maker, a singer, a painter, a player, and so on. The essence refers to the core of mankind, what makes man really human.

I agree with Van der Klis that this way of reasoning raises many questions. First, when everybody claims that his medium of art is the essence of life, there seem to be many essences. Can there be several essences? Second, the essence put forward mostly is deduced from a stage of development in human life. However, does it make any sense to say that what comes first in development is the essence of life? For example, should we conclude that because a fetus first develops touch and the sense of equilibrium, these are more essential than hearing and seeing? Third, is it appropriate to make arts therapies trustworthy because the medium is connected to early phases of development? This only makes sense when disturbances and handicaps are linked to a particular phase of development, and should be cured by means of regression.

By the *holistic* trap of reasoning, Van der Klis refers to the idea that everything influences everything. I do not want to criticize the idea of holism as such. What I want to question is the form of simplistic holistic reasoning that states that arts therapies are indicated for each client, because arts therapies result in a change in creativity that inevitably changes the whole person, and thus the disturbance. This type of reasoning is axiomatic and almost magical, but unable to answer the question of why, for example, music therapy is indicated for depression. In my opinion, in this example, it should be clear that music therapy stimulates those personal processes a depressed person needs to overcome his depression, and why.

The Need for Client-Centered Indications

Van Audenhove (1995), a psychotherapist, mentions a lack of attunement of the client's needs and the supplies clinics can offer. A client does not get what he needs, but what a clinic provides. Instead of selecting a psychotherapeutic method that is most appropriate, a client is treated by the psychotherapeutic method the clinic has decided upon beforehand.

The same holds true for the arts therapies. I discussed before the situation where a music therapist is forced to develop a method, and then it is asked, "Who is the right client for music therapy?" Clients often are referred to a specific type of art therapy because it is there, not because it is most appropriate for the client's needs.

To match arts therapies to the client's need, there should be an exchange between the arts therapists, who inform the client about appropriate possibilities for treatment, and the client himself, who knows his needs and from his perspective will be able to decide if the offered possibilities are coherent with his needs.

Working in Multidisciplinary Teams

Verhey (1997) points out that indications for arts therapies should be part of multidisciplinary consultation. Arts therapists should bring their assessment results to the multidisciplinary team, and together with the other members of the team develop a diagnosis, map out treatment goals, and decide which methods are appropriate to reach these goals.

The arts therapists, on the one hand, should contribute to the total treatment plan; on the other hand, they should inform colleagues from other professions what arts therapies can add to the treatment goals. The multidisciplinary team should discuss who among it is able to do what and able to do it best.

EPILOGUE: A CLIENT-FOCUSED AND EVIDENCE-BASED MUSIC THERAPY TREATMENT

The criteria for indications can help the music therapists (and the arts therapists in general) to avoid the trap of essentialism and holism. They will enable them to give information about possibilities and effects of the treatment to their clients, and will also give them a scientific background to advocate their treatment in the multidisciplinary team. It is important that indications become adjusted to the areas of treatment. Whether music therapy (or another type of art therapy) is indicated strongly depends on the client group.

Discussion groups of music therapists and researchers working with the same client group can make explicit tacit knowledge, develop consensus-based best practices, and adjust treatment by including research results. Then there will be client-focused and evidence-based treatment.

Chapter Three

TOWARD A GENERAL THEORY OF MUSIC THERAPY?

INTRODUCTION

During the 4th European Music Therapy Conference in Leuven (1998), a discussion about the possibility of developing a general theory of music therapy began. A dialogue between Carolyn Kenny and me preceded this discussion. Colleagues were invited to take part in a process of "peer debriefing."[5]

In this chapter, I will describe some core questions that came up in the dialogue and process of peer debriefing. I will focus on questions that come forward if you want to develop a general theory of music therapy. In Part II of this book, I will develop the theory of analogy, which perhaps might be a "general theory" of music therapy in the sense that it gives a general explanation of the question why music therapy works.

Before developing this theory, I would like to reflect on the critical aspects of my own attempt.

THE DIALOGUE

Introduction

This dialogue is a follow-up to the discussion on theory development. Science grows by means of multiple perspectives, which should be developed and accepted not as conflicting views, but as complementary ones. I take some of the

---

[5]Carolyn Kenny and I had initiated this discussion. David Aldridge, Dorit Amir, Lars Ole Bonde, Kimmo Lehtonen, Wolfgang Mahns, Mercedes Pavlicevic, Brynjulf Stige, Eckard Weymann, Kenneth Aigen, Diane Austin, and Even Ruud gave written or verbal comments during the Leuven seminar. Since then, this discussion has been continued in *Voices: A World Forum for Music Therapy* and in journals such as the *Nordic Journal of Music Therapy* (see, for instance, the discussion between Bärmark, Hallin, Garred, and Kenny and the series "Theory Building in Music Therapy--An International Archive").

central issues in Kenny's perspective and elaborate on them. As you will see, there will be agreements as well as differences.

When I discussed Kenny's contribution to qualitative research in my book on qualitative research (*Multiple perspectives: A guide to qualitative research in music therapy*, 1997b), this brought me back to basic questions such as, "What is knowledge?" "What do we know?" "What can we know?" These same questions are basic to this chapter.

What Can Theory Offer Us?

Several music therapists do not believe that a general theory is possible. Stige (1999), for instance, while referring to Wittgenstein, concludes that the variety within music therapy cannot be captured in one general theory. Meaning, he says, can only be related to a specific context, and knowledge cannot be context independent. Herewith he raises the paradox between the general theory and local theories, and the question of whether a general theory can be developed that will be able to include the local theories. Perhaps we should ask ourselves which meaning can be general and which meaning should be local. When local meaning is confused with general meaning, we get in trouble. For example, the meaning a client gives to music is personal, and thus it is impossible to declare that a particular piece of music will have the same effect on different clients. However, this does not mean that there are no general meanings about music therapy possible. The point is that a general theory should not be based on those meanings that can only be local.

Kenny calls immediacy one of the critical factors of the effectiveness of music therapy. When we take this immediacy seriously, then this has consequences for theorizing, because theory is not immediate. Theory is abstract and digital; it offers codes that are distanced from the phenomena they refer to.

Kenny is telling us explicitly that her memory is full of hundreds of clients. She wants to be close to her experiences as a music therapist, those experiences that give her immediate knowledge. Kenny uses "just enough" abstract thinking to make theory possible (Kenny, 1997)--no less and (what is most important) no more. If you push theory too far, you get dragons (Kenny, 1999).

When an experience itself is immediate and not distanced, how then can we theorize about it? Is it possible to describe in words and concepts the immediate musical experience, which in itself is beyond words? Using the word "immediate" in a theoretical model does not imply that we "understand" immediacy. Coding the experience means knowing that it is there, but this is not the same as knowing the experience.

There also is a problem of research methodology. If we need to experience immediacy to "know" what it is, then the consequence would be that they who are in the immediacy of the musical experience, the music therapists and clients, are the ones who should develop theories. But even then, they are confronted with the problem of communicating their theory, which is grounded in the immediate experience, to others. Will others ever be able to understand the music therapist's and client's codes if they themselves never have been in the same experience?

Perhaps we should introduce the guideline that researchers who want to understand music therapy must go into the music therapy experience themselves, to know by experience what it is. But even this guideline will not make it possible to replicate the same experience.

During the past few years, it has become evident that journals should not only write about music therapy, but also include the music. It also became evident that qualitative narratives are more adequate to describe musical experiences. By doing this, it perhaps will be possible for an outsider to be in contact with the immediate experiences more directly. But nevertheless, it will be difficult to understand the immediate experience in the music that unfolds between the client and the music therapist.

We might ask ourselves whether this particular problem is a problem only for music therapy. Perhaps it is a much more fundamental problem of knowledge. Let me quote a Dutch behavioral therapist who advocates behavioral therapy by saying that pure knowledge has less influence than knowing by experience. Knowing a citron is very different from biting into it, he says (Orlemans, 1994). Although this sentence perhaps seems surprising for a behaviorist, because it refers to an inner experience, it contains an important truth. Tasting a citron, smelling a flower, listening to the vitality affects of someone's psyche, is different from reading verbal codes.

In the example of the citron, we are able to "know" the citron, because we once have been in the experience of eating a citron ourselves, and anytime can go into the experience again. In this case the problem of research methodology has been solved: Each researcher can replicate the experience of the citron. Thus, when he develops a theory about the citron, his codes are grounded in the known experience.

To understand experiences that have been put into words, the words have to be decoded. Perhaps it is a disadvantage of mankind to be a symbolizing species, because whenever experiences have been coded in words, there is the risk that experiences get lost. What results is that instead of sharing experiences, persons talk about experiences. Then the theory about phenomena is distanced from experiencing the phenomena.

We should make two objections here and take into account that, first, using words in itself is an experience, and, second, words from authors and poets can evoke deep experiences. This brings us to a seeming paradox of directness.

Mystery Instead of Theory?

When Kenny discusses empathy, she focuses on the empathy of the music therapist for the client. She puts forward that in the case of empathy, when there is theorizing, there is a distance from the experience of empathy. Again, we can ask how the experience of empathy, which is immediate, can be put into a theory. How can the experience of empathy, which in itself is beyond words, be described in words?

Kenny introduces the word mystery, and tells us that we remove from experience because we are afraid of mysterious experiences that cannot be described in words. I would like to add that we escape from what cannot be described into some-thing that can be described. But this some-thing is different from the authentic experience.

However, I hesitate to use the word mystery. In the first place, I do not advocate words such as mystery, because I think that we should try to develop a theory with concepts that are less spiritual. A second reason is that a word such as mystery may obscure music therapy. A person who does not know the experience, who is not able to theorize on the basis of experiences, can use the same word. In other words, the nonprofessional can call himself a professional by saying that what he is doing is a mystery, about which he is unable to speak. A third reason is that in the professional health care system nowadays, it is very difficult to validate music therapy by using words such as mystery.

On the other hand, perhaps we indeed should be less afraid of the mystery that takes place in personal encounters. The word mystery is comparable to Sartre's concept of Le Néant, telling us that man cannot be described as *some-thing*, but only as not-some-thing, *no*-thing. The empathic experience in music therapy cannot exactly be interpreted and described in words either. Therefore the word mystery—which is a word--points to *this being beyond words*, the no-word, no-theory dimension of (intra- and interpersonal) experience.

Uniqueness

I said before that when we escape into *some-thing* that can be described, this some-thing differs from the experience we want to describe. When discussing the difference between quantitative and qualitative research in the *Multiple Perspectives* book, I summarized the quantitative paradigm by saying that it makes it possible to research "some-thing" (a mean score of an excerpt of behavior). However, a reality that is reduced by measuring instruments and pre-established theory cannot reconstruct the naturalistic situation, nor the unique persons and their experiences herein.

Horkheimer and Adorno, in their *Dialektik der Aufklärung* (1981), describe how language and science have become tools to control "things," and how "truth" has been identified with the positivistic scientific manipulative techniques.

As Horkheimer and Adorno point out, positivistic methodology violates the unfamiliar. Kenny tells us that positivistic science when measuring the *some-thing* focuses on isolated common aspects, violating the unfamiliar and thus the unique wholeness. Phenomena become some-things that can be known by positivistic science. The choice between the unique and the standardized is a choice of paradigm, which is connected to the research focus. The choice a researcher makes cannot be proved, but comes from his personal life philosophy. Therefore, there is no value-free science.

These thoughts gave way to two conclusions. The first conclusion states that research can focus on standardization because in life there is standardization, too. The second conclusion is that what really counts in personal life is the difference. What is really important for a human being is his being different from anybody else, his uniqueness. The therapist's aim is "making special" (Kenny, quoting Dissanayake). There is nobody like me and there is nobody like you.

The uniqueness again puts forward the question of what theory can offer us. Theorizing means developing concepts that are meant to be universal. Is it possible to develop universal concepts that make possible uniqueness? Can there be a general theory that is flexible and fluid (Kenny)? Will we be able to develop universal concepts that give structure to flexible and fluid contents? These universal concepts must be able to refer to the music therapy treatment of many disturbances and handicaps and to the big landscape of music therapy methods. As we shall see in Chapter Five, these questions will guide the development of the theory of analogy.

The Dilemma of Music Therapy

What really counts in personal life is the uniqueness of human beings. However, in life there is standardization, too. Several psychotherapeutic schools have been developed that focus on this uniqueness, advocating methods of therapy and research that are nonstandardized. On the contrary, the (neo)positivistic paradigm focuses on the standardized.

It is somehow difficult to explain cause and effect in the history of therapy and research. Was there first the opinion that therapy should focus on the shared characteristics of mankind, which led to the development of the positivistic research methodology that makes it possible to research these shared characteristics? Or was it the other way around, and did it all start with the opinion that therapy should focus on the shared characteristics of mankind, because these can be researched by positivistic research?

In any case, nowadays the positivistic research methodology is advocated as the toughest research. It seems as if we are not allowed to talk about what cannot be researched in a positivistic way. The axiom of this point of view is that only one particular research methodology (the positivistic) is trustworthy. It brings music therapy (and other therapies) into a vulnerable dilemma.

I think that we should solve the dilemma by using both research paradigms. What really counts is the uniqueness, but what man encounters can be shared.

PEER DEBRIEFING

In this section, I will highlight several important comments that have been made by members of the expert panel who took part in the process of "peer debriefing." In general, there was approval and support for the attempt to develop a general theory of music therapy. However, all members of the panel put forward critical issues.[6] There also was some frustration. One of the panel members discussed the paper with his students, who felt discouraged because they experienced the theoretical model as "too big."

Now let me summarize three important comments by the panel members[7]: one about the dilemma of generality, one about what is reflected in the music, and one about improvement.

General Theory

One of the most important considerations of the panel members was that general theory should respect diversity, and that theory should not become too simplistic and too universal. One of the panel members called the intention to create a general theory a little bit "vulgar." These comments illustrate once more the fundamental issue of whether a general theory is possible, and what the advantages and disadvantages of such a theory would be. The panel members illuminate the dilemma of the general and the specific. There is discontent about generalization, about distancing from the "local theory," from the particular and local, about losing contact with the diversity and deepness of the experience. Several panel members claimed that theory should be grounded in the local, and that we need many theories for many clients. A shared conceptual system can

---

[6]In this chapter, I will focus on comments about theory in general. Comments about the theory of analogy will be included in the epilogue of the book.

[7]These were individual comments and not consensus-based comments. I made a cross-analysis of all individual comments.

stimulate communication and thus professionalization, but it also can obstruct the view of the special.

On the other hand, the comments show that a need is felt for some rigor of thinking. I certainly agree with this. I think that we need to exchange our ideas and try to establish some basic agreement about music therapy. In my opinion, the schools of music therapy, until now, have been developed in isolation too much. The time has come to research the nonspecific shared characteristics of different models of music therapy. I am convinced that from the clinical work of music therapists with different theoretical backgrounds, we can deduce sensitizing concepts and core categories. The need for local theories for individual clients cannot release us from the obligation to research the nonspecific factors of these local theories.

From the comments, we can conclude that we need a discussion about what a theory should look like. As a central question, we need to ask ourselves how a theory of music therapy can connect the universal and special.

Sounding the Therapeutic Relationship

Two interesting points made by panel members were about re-sounding and the therapeutic relationship. In my discussion paper, I talked about re-sounding (instead of reflecting) the client's psyche in the music. By replacing reflecting with re-sounding, I want to stress that the client "shows" himself in musical sounds. Re-sounding meant to describe the "mirror of sounds."

Some panel members thought that music therapy is not *re-sounding*, *re-creating*, *repeating*, or *re-exploring* aspects of the client's life, but *sounding* his life in the here-and-now. I agree with this, because when I introduced the term "re-sounding," I did not mean that the client is repeating some experience from the past, but that he sounds his or her own Self in the here-and-now, which of course can include here-and-now experiences of past experiences.

A second comment was that music therapy is not about sounding the client's inner psyche in the music, but about sounding the relationship between client and music therapist. This shows that some panel members were convinced that it is not the music that heals, but the therapeutic relationship.

I cannot agree fully with this. Of course, the sounding includes the therapeutic relationship, but I am not convinced that it is the therapeutic relationship only that is the therapeutic mover. I think that the sounding of intra- and interpersonal phenomena in the music is what gives music therapy its therapeutic power.

Making Special

Another idea that was challenged during peer debriefing was my point of view that the goal of music therapy is "to change." It was brought to the fore that maybe the goal of music therapy is not "to change," but to "make special" the client's world (see Kenny, 1996b). By reacting with empathy, the client's world becomes "special--to someone else." The therapeutic transformation might simply be that another shares the client's world.

This comment is fundamental not only to music therapy but to all sorts of therapy. It can be based on different paradigms. One paradigm is more existential-humanistic; another is more technical in character. The former tells us that therapists think that clients improve because they do not want to be treated as a sample; the latter states that therapists think that clients improve because they know that treating them as a sample is something the therapist knows how to handle. Maybe both perspectives are credible, depending on the therapist's and client's own views, which can be constructed in the therapeutic alliance. One client may improve when he feels he is special; another client may improve when he thinks he receives care that has been tried out in similar cases.

In any case, the client is helped by the therapist to go into experiences that make it possible that he experiences something different in his being-in-the-world. As one of the panel members wrote, in music therapy change can occur because the music contains more meaning than therapist and client have put into it. Because of this extended meaning, the client has the opportunity to travel into different areas of experience.

Although these comments are limited, they illustrate that when developing a theory of music therapy, answers have to be found about its universality, what it is that is sounded in the music, why music therapy works, and what its goal is. Even a limited process of peer debriefing immediately pops up with several essential questions a theory of music therapy needs to cover.

In the epilogue of this book, I will continue these comments and focus on topics in the discussion that were connected to the theory of analogy.

A CATEGORIZATION OF QUESTIONS AND STATEMENTS

In this section, I will formulate questions and statements that we should have in our mind when developing a general theory of music therapy. These questions are a result of the cross-analysis I carried out on the individual comments of the panel members. Table 3.1 shows questions and statements of the panel members, structured into categories.

Table 3.1
Categories About General Theory

About the Benefit of a General Theory

- Why should we develop a general theory?
- Can a general theory be useful?
- Who is going to use a general theory?
- Can a general theory be misused?

About the Structure of a General Theory

- What should a general theory look like?
- What types of universalities can be included in a general theory?
- Can there be consensus about universalities?
- How can a general theory include multiple perspectives?

About Universality and Uniqueness

- How can a general theory include multiple perspectives?
- How can we theorize about immediate experiences?
- How can we manage the dilemma of universality and uniqueness, of the repetitive and nonrepetitive, of sampling and making special?
- Will a general theory be able to deal with the complexity of experience?
- Should we develop many particular local theories?
- Is it possible to describe universal basic processes that are fundamental to many realities?
- Should theory come from practice completely or should we make use of other theoretical perspectives?
- Is there a risk that other theoretical perspectives will be superimposed on the music therapy experiences?
- Should we accept that theory is always different from immediate experiences?

About the Language of a General Theory

- Which types of verbal codes should be used?
- How can we connect musical and psychological concepts?
- How can we deal with the dilemma of a verbal theory and the nonverbal experiences in music therapy?
- Can music therapists and clients understand a general theory?
- Should we develop several languages for several levels of dialogue?

About Researching General Theory

- Which research paradigm is needed to generate a general theory?
- How can we manage the feedback loop of deconstructing and constructing?
- Should music therapists and clients research music therapy?
- Should researchers who want to understand music therapy go into music therapy experience themselves?

About Music and Language

- Is it allowable to say that music is "in" the experience and language is "about" the experience?
- Is there a difference between the "embodied" meaning of music and words?
- Should we say that music offers a way out of verbal reality?

As we all know, there are more questions than answers. Nevertheless, let these (and other) questions be landmarks for everyone who wants to develop a theory of music therapy.

PART II:

TOWARD A THEORY OF ANALOGY IN MUSIC THERAPY

Chapter Four

THE POWER OF MUSIC

INTRODUCTION

The observation by Vincent van Gogh that he did not paint what he saw, but indeed what he felt, in the work of George Steiner (1968), has been turned into a revolutionary conclusion. What we see, Steiner says, can be put into words; what we feel precedes language or goes beyond it.

Steiner thinks that music is the most important language that is able to express feeling. What does he mean, and how can we understand this conclusion, knowing that every painter and author will strongly oppose it? There is a rich historical collection of poems and novels—all made of words—by which a lot of feelings can be aroused. And what about painting? Why quote Vincent van Gogh and then conclude that music is the most important art? Is Steiner serious?

FORM AND CONTENT

Steiner makes an exception for poems, which in his opinion come close to music. He quotes Paul Verlaine's principle—"De la musique avant toute chose"—and explains that in a poem, sound is more important than notion. But even if we agree with Steiner that "poetry leads to music," there still are the novels that can evoke many feelings. Steiner proceeds by saying that in music—not in painting and writing—there is a complete melting of form and content. Therefore, as Thomas Mann put it, "The composer is the artist par excellence."

This brings us to the question of form and content, a question with a heavy historical load. Before further exploring this question, we should remember that there is music where this equalization of form and content does not hold because there is some "content" outside the music (for instance, in operas), and that on the contrary there are paintings where there is no content "out there" and form is content (for such as, abstract paintings).

Now let us try to explore what it means to say that form is content and content is form. Steiner uses a very trivial example. In his opinion, someone who is tired easily can listen even to complex music, but will be unable to read a novel. The brain, Steiner says, is not confused by music.

We should not take this as a neurological statement but as Steiner's own experience. Perhaps it could be explained from Steiner's own personal background, being a professor of literature who after hours of reading relaxes by listening to music. When we try to generalize Steiner's statement, it becomes clear that it is only partly true. As we know from music psychology research, listening strategies of people can be very different. Some people prefer listening to complex music; others prefer music that is less complex. What is more, the listening strategy of one person can change from day to day, depending on his mood (for a review of these findings, see Smeijsters, 1995/1999b). For instance, if you like Mahler symphonies, this does not mean that when you are tired from work you will listen to one. Can there be some "truth" in Steiner's claim?

COGNITIVE PROCESSING

Imagine reading a novel. In any case, your mind needs to make some use of "interpretation." You cannot just read the words one after another without any cognitive activity. You need to remember (Who is who? What are their characteristics? Who is doing what?), associate (connect somebody's behavior to the behavior of somebody else), imagine (imagine what the persons, circumstances, and events look like), think (What does it mean? Where does this lead to?), and so on. A novel always has a plot that we need to reconstruct in our mind. The words refer to this plot; they are intermediary objects that make possible the creation of an event in our mind. If there is no cognitive knowledge when reading a novel, we cannot make any sense out of it, and the novel has "no meaning." Without this cognitive activity, there is only the rhythm of word accents, which perhaps reminds you of music.

Music can be understood even when there is no such cognitive knowledge. Everybody can listen to and "understand" Beethoven symphonies, but not everybody can understand Thomas Mann's *Dokter Faustus* or Hermann Broch's *Der Tod des Vergil.* Of course, they can "read" the words, but they cannot understand the plot, and thus reading makes no sense.

Although music by the composer is cognitively constructed equal to the way a novel is constructed by its author, listening to music is different from reading a novel. I am not talking about the professional literature critique that discusses from a scientific perspective how the novel is organized, nor am I pointing to the professional music theorist who makes a musical analysis. I am talking about the nonscientific reader and the nontheoretical listener, and maintaining that in this case reading is different from listening.

There seem to be two kinds of "knowledge" then. One type makes use of a cognitive (secondary) process. If this process unfolds, then other spheres of human life, such as feeling, can be evoked. Music does not need this secondary type of knowledge. Musical sounds do not "refer"; there are no "intermediary objects." Music is something "in itself," not referring to something else but resting in itself. Although a listener can try to remember and to predict, these processes are different because music is remembered and predicted in itself; there is no "plot" outside the sounds as there is outside the words. Music has "meaning," even if it has no referential meaning. We can conclude from this that music and novels belong to different types of knowledge.

MUSIC: THE IRRATIONAL AND NUMINOUS

The power of music is that it goes directly into our world of feelings without the need of an intermediary process of remembering, thinking, associating, and imagining. There is no need for such a secondary cognitive process to "understand" music, to feel that it is about you. There is no "story" we recognize as having any connection with our life perspective. There only are sounds, and we are strongly moved by them. In Steiner's view, because of this, music is "irrational." We are moved by it although we do not know what it is all about.

The power of music makes it even "numinous"; we are attracted by it and at the same time experience fear. There is something personal that is beyond our command. Music brings us to layers of our experience that can be experienced but cannot be put into words, and it sounds the preconscious, subconscious, and unconscious layers of our psyche. This explains Ionesco's words, quoted by Steiner: "The more I try to explain myself by words, the less I understand myself. Not everything is beyond words, but the living truth is."

But still there are many questions. Steiner's revelations such as "Music is the source of the pure," "Music is more deep and more comprehensive than language," "Music directly sprouts from the sources of our being," and "The question 'What is music?' is the same question as 'What is mankind?'"; his quotations from artists such as Thomas Mann, Eugène Ionesco, and Rainer Maria Rilke; and his examples from *La Devina Commedia* and *Moses und Aron,* where words fail to give the imagination, still are not a real answer to the question of why music has this power. The examples are expressive and render account of the fact that authors feel the impotence of words, but we need a more psychomusicological understanding of this matter.

Before I focus more deeply on the nonreferential aspect of music, I want to make some comments about music therapy. If we take seriously what has been said previously, then going into the music for the client means being attracted by it and experiencing fear also. Going into the improvisation in music therapy is ominous. Music bypasses the rational. It is this irrational aspect which gives music its healing power. Clients live in an irrational world where words have no access, or in a rational world where they are imprisoned by words. Music is a means to enter the irrational world and to bypass the overrationalized world.

When Steiner asserts that in today's world too many books are written, that there is too much and too easy small talk, that there should be more "silence," I am not sure whether this is different for music. In today's world, we have too much background music in shops, stations, and airports. Even in health institutions, music never stops. To be healing, music should be personal, and the client needs a music therapist who can help in exploring the client's psyche in the music.

REFERENTIAL MEANING OF 'EMPTY' WORDS

Steiner claims that verbal language is impoverished. This impoverishment is an impoverishment of meaning. In his opinion, the meaning of words has been corrupted by military undertakings and advertisements. Indeed, we are forced to believe that there can be a "clean" war and that an aftershave can make us "happy."

The problem with verbal language seems to be that each word implies something to which it refers. If this "something" is operationalized, then the meaning becomes clear-cut, and the rich, authentic, unspecified meaning has been lost. I suggest that the power of music comes from the fact that its meaning is not operationalized, because we do not try to grasp the meaning of music, which would be gone if we tried to grasp it. Words become less pure because they are filled with meaning. When there is no meaning, as in sounds, this meaning cannot become corrupted.

It is difficult to convince another person by means of words that you share his feelings. Many times words are inadequate because they are just labels that easily can be spoken while the empathic feeling itself needs a distinct medium of expression. As Steiner puts it, "There is a tragic gap between what can be understood and what can be said. Words twist, eloquent words twist absolute." I think that clients feel strongly that felt knowledge and acceptance is beyond words.[1] Many clients became sick of this lack of real understanding.

The word "rose," Steiner explicates, is an empty phonetic marker; it has nothing to do with the rose, as such, to which it points. There is no correspondence between the word and the real thing. The word rose is not red.

---

[1]This resembles Stern's opinion about literal imitation versus cross-modal answers (Stern, 1985). If someone reacts by doing exactly the same as I did, I feel that he is like a mirror, but can I infer from this that he feels the same?

We can only experience what a rose is by looking at it and smelling it. If we use words to talk about the rose, our real experience of the rose is lost, or is only memory. The more we use words to talk about things, the less we experience the real things. What we get is a "world of words," which is distinct from the real world. We are forcing ourselves into the dualism of the objects and the world of words that points to the objects.

This reminds me of those people who "know" what has been written about phenomena, but are unable to experience these phenomena themselves. This is very detrimental in therapy, training, and research. A therapist cannot "understand" his client by precoding him along theoretical lines. Only a personal encounter where the client is experienced as an individual person leads to real knowledge. Perhaps afterwards it can be concluded that some of the experiences are similar to theoretical concepts. The same holds true for the training process, where students should not be forced into theories that take over their personal experiences, and for research, where researchers should be "open" to experience and to experience themselves what they are researching. Although a researcher will have to use words, being in the experience himself at least ensures that the words are "grounded" in real experiences. Theories give power, just as words are powerful tools to organize the world. But theories, like words, become destructive weapons when they replace the authentic personal experience and engagement.

Steiner's "empty" meaning of words in the psychology of communication has been conceptualized as "digital" versus "analogous" communication. Like the digital language of computers, words have no resemblance to what they mean. They are "empty." What about music then?

In this book, I will explain how musical processes are analogies of psychological processes. As I said before, musical sounds do not "refer" to something; musical sounds exist "in themselves." But at the same time, they are not "empty." Although they are not referring to something, they "are" something. This seems to be a paradox because when musical sounds are something, we think they should refer to something. But the point is that when you express yourself in musical sounds, you are the sounds and the sounds are you. When your sounds are quiet, you are quiet; when your sounds are quick, you are quick. When your sounds are strong, you are strong; when there is discontinuity in the sounds, there is discontinuity in you. The sounds do not refer to you. They do not tell something about you, but they are you. You and the musical sounds are "equal."

SYMBOLIC KNOWLEDGE

A word is a symbol. There are other types of symbols, which, like words, can refer to something without resembling it. The symbol acts as a reference to something, and therefore it is "indirect." A metaphor is "indirect," too. It takes something else's meaning and combines it with something new to give more knowledge to the new. By means of interpretation, it can be concluded that the new thing is "like" the other. Both symbol and metaphor take things from outside to refer to or interpret the thing itself.

Now I want to research more deeply the difference between the "indirect" and the "direct" knowledge. Wilber (1987) quotes Eddington when distinguishing between two ways of knowledge. The first, Eddington says, is "symbolic knowledge"; the second one is "intimate knowledge."

Symbolic knowledge works by coding and analyzing. When we, by means of symbols, code and analyze, the intimacy of the experience is replaced. We are not in the experience anymore, but separated from it; there is no more directness, but indirectness. Wilber defines symbolic meaning as "dualistic": The symbol is separated from the thing it represents. Symbolic knowledge is a substitution for intimate knowledge.

In symbolic knowledge, there is an experience and something outside the experience that gives a name and a meaning to the experience. There is a representation, which can be useful—but still it is a representation. The representation is somehow artificial, as plastic flowers represent real flowers very well but are not real flowers. For some people, this difference does not matter; for example, many people think that talking about experience is just like experiencing.[2] But, as Wilber states, "The word 'heaven' is not blue, and the word 'water' cannot quench your thirst." Remember Steiner's example of the word rose, which is not red.

Symbolic knowledge is knowledge "about," not knowledge "in." Steiner calls to question all those literature critics who try to understand works of art by writing "about" them, but do not understand art by producing works of art themselves. Steiner's argument is that to understand art, you must be an artist and make works of art yourself.

Whitehead, quoted by Wilber, sees symbolizing as an act of abstracting where only certain characteristics come to the fore and others are ignored. But notwithstanding this, people conceive the abstractions as the concrete realities. It is like prejudice, when people are abstracted as a member of a social group and the supposed characteristics of the social group are applied to the unique person. In the quantitative research paradigm, complexity is reduced to variables, which

[2]Talking is an experience in itself, but when you talk about another experience, this talking about is different from the primary experience.

are believed to predict complexity. Intimate knowledge, on the contrary, is intuitive, nonintermediary, nonsubstitutional, nondualistic, direct, and nonabstract.

Within symbolic knowledge, Wilber differentiates two types: the "linear, one-dimensional, analytic, and logical" one, and the "imaginative, more-dimensional, artistic, dream-oriented, nonlogical" one. From these two types of symbolic knowledge, he deduces three ways to "talk about spirit."

In his definition, the *analogous* representation ascribes properties to reality that give an idea of the "absolute," such as "omnipotence," "omnipresence," "omniscience," "highest blessing," "highest wisdom and love." Wilber defines these descriptions as linear but also imaginative when supplemented by symbols, such as the holy cross, and myths, such as the bible.

The *negative* representation is like creating a sculpture in which all parts that are disturbing are eliminated. Then the "absolute" is "not this," and "not that." In the opinion of Wilber, both the analogous and the negative type of representation are "small talks," useless attempts to define what cannot be defined.

The third, *injunctive,* way of representing gives a set of rules that have to be followed if someone wants to uncover reality. The rules point in a direction, but do not coincide with its destination. As in baking, there is a recipe that produces a cake if you follow the directions. Wilber gives also the example of the composer who in the musical score gives instructions on how to reproduce his original musical experience.

According to Wilber, the analogous, negative, and injunctive ways tell you "how" reality is, what it "is not," and what you can do to experience it; they do not tell us what reality "is." I would like to discuss some of my basic thoughts that differ from those of Wilber. First, in my opinion musical "knowledge" is different from Wilber's second—imaginative—type of symbolic knowledge. The imaginative symbolic knowledge is indeed different from the logical symbolism in the first type of symbolic knowledge. Like dreams, it depends on images, which refer to meaningful experiences that are difficult to grasp. The point is that symbolic images point to meaningful experiences. Music is different from such a symbolic image. The meaning of music is embodied meaning. In music, form and content (the meaning) are not separated. Musical form conforms to the meaningful experience.[3]

Imagine yourself being part of a musical improvisation. You are playing and joining rhythms, tempi, dynamics, melodies, and harmonies, which develop as processes and all together make a musical form. These processes have

---

[3]One should distinguish between images (such as a cross or a color) that refer to meaningful content, and images—such as the images produced in art therapy—which, like music, may have meaning embodied in their structure.

"meaning," not in a symbolic referential, but in a direct, immediate way. The musical processes conform to the basic processes of the inner psyche and the interpersonal life. These processes need no translation into images because the musical processes "sound" intra- and interpersonal processes.[4] Because musical meaning is embodied meaning, musical knowledge is different from knowledge that is transmitted through images, and music should not be translated into images.

Second, my opinion about analogy differs from what Wilber describes as analogous. In his opinion, the analogous representation uses words, symbolic images, and myths that give an idea of what reality is. This, in my opinion, is not an analogy, because there is no resemblance between a word such as "omnipotence," the cross, and the religious experience of reality. What Wilber has called analogous representation has been researched in music therapy. Although it certainly is helpful to describe by means of words the meaningful moments people experience in music therapy (see Amir, 1996), these words are not analogies of the experiences.[5]

Third, Wilber describes the specific role of music when he gives the example of the composer and when he categorizes music as injunctive representation. And, of course, in musical improvisation there can be rules that bring us into a process. The example of baking shows that he distinguishes between the process, which is guided by rules, and the final product, the cake. But in musical improvisation there is no dichotomy of process and product. The musical improvisation is the product, and by being in the process, the improviser is "in" the experience.

INTIMATE KNOWLEDGE

Carolyn Kenny, in her book *The Field of Play* (1989), states that "... we must be doing, or at least vividly remembering, music therapy experience while designing philosophy and theory" (p. 47). Central to her statement is the "music therapy experience" and how to replicate it. The first possibility for replicating,

---

[4]Instead of "reflect" I use the word "sound" to state that in music therapy experiences are made in sound and not in images. I use "sound" instead of "re-sound" to state that music therapy is not about repeating experiences in sound, but about sound experiences in the here-and-now (with thanks to Mercedes Pavlicevic for her comment on this).

[5]Amir, in her research on meaningful moments, gives examples of impressive experiences such as awareness, acceptance, freedom, wholeness, completion, beauty, inner transformation, spirituality, intimacy, ecstasy, and so on.

Kenny suggests, is by doing. The second possibility she gives is to vividly remember the experience. Her words "at least" tell us that the second solution is not as good as the first one. In any case, there must have been an original experience in the past that we can remember in our mind vividly as and if it happens again.

In both possibilities—doing or remembering—we experience, de facto or in our imagination. We are not referring to experience, but we are in the experience itself. Kenny uses words such as "direct" and "immediate," and quotes Polanyi, who claimed that there is no knowledge outside experience. Kenny puts forward that music is "a language of immediacy."

Whether we agree with Polanyi's statement that there is no knowledge outside experience depends on what we define as "knowledge." In the previous section, I distinguished between two types of "knowledge." One type makes use of symbols that tell us something "about" an experience; the other type is nonsymbolic, and is embodied in the experience itself. Human beings are able to mentally play with symbols, which represents the first type of knowledge. The second type of knowledge, the "intimate" knowledge, cannot exist outside experience. This knowledge is defined as "what is in the experience."

Because of its nonsymbolic character, its embodied meaning, its unity of form and content, music makes possible intimate knowledge. Being in the music is being in the experience. Kenny states that it is the direct experience of sensations in art that leads to consciousness (knowledge). There are two strong points in this statement. The first is that by mentioning sensations it becomes clear where "directness" comes from. The second strong point is that this puts forward art, because it is art that gives us sensations. Thus, Kenny tells us that we need to be close to direct experiences, sensations give us direct experiences, art gives us sensations, and thus art gives us direct experiences.

There are two points in her line of thought that need further discussion. First, I think that we need to go beyond sensations, because the consciousness of sensations gives only a limited "sensualistic" definition of consciousness. We should look for a bridge between sensations and psychological phenomena, which will be able to explain why arts therapies can cure psychological disturbances. Second, we should specify music more closely. I would like to describe the musical characteristics. Although I agree with Kenny's statement that music is a language of immediate experience, I want to know what this immediate experience is.

When music indeed gives us direct experience, then perhaps we should claim that the "musical method" is more valid than any method of scientific research that translates experience into symbols (words and figures). By bringing the client into the music and sharing the music with him, both client and music therapist reach immediate knowledge.

Why do we need a research method that describes in a dualistic way experiences, when being in the music gives us the intimate knowledge of experiences? Why should we exchange immediate knowledge for intermediate knowledge?

If we take these questions seriously, we need a paradigm shift that leads to science using sounds instead of words (other researchers in the arts therapies advocate this position; see Langenberg, Aigen & Frommer, 1996; McNiff, 1998; Grainger, 1999, 2001/02. It might imply that the music therapist and the client meet each other in the music, that they decrease the amount of talking about their experiences, and that the music therapist does write fewer articles about it. The music therapist would say to his client and to his colleagues, "Listen to the sound." This would be very close to Steiner's example of Robert Schumann, who, when asked to explain a piece of music, instead of talking about it, sat behind the piano and played the piece. In Steiner's opinion, music is "irreducible"; it cannot be explained by "small talk." We now might add that experience in music therapy is irreducible—it cannot be described by words. What can be described by words is the symbolic type of knowledge, which is "about" experience, but not experience itself.

Let me give you one final quotation of Wilber (1987): "All judgments and thoughts about reality are empty and insignificant ... reality cannot be represented, but it can be experienced" (p. 86). As you can see from the following quotations, an experienced music therapist such as Kenny shares this idea: "I cannot compromise these moments (in music therapy), which represented hundreds of other patients and clients over 25 years of practice, with language that is a lie. ... These were moments of intense beauty in a heightened state of awareness. In a sense, they are beyond words" (Kenny, 1996b, p. 73). And: "What we know is in the music, in the sound. At least that's the way it is for me. Other things come second, including cognizing" (Kenny, 1996a, p. 197). Improvisation in music therapy is an event in reality that makes reality experiential. Its experiential meaning cannot be represented by words.

CONCLUSIONS AND OUTLOOK

I think that it is important to be aware that it is very difficult to understand someone else's experience when you never have been in the same experience. Are we ever able to share the feelings of someone who has been sexually abused, of someone who has been traumatized because of an accident, of someone who has become schizophrenic? As Kenny (1996b, p. 63) says, "Can I comment on the worldview of the patient with confidence? The answer is no." Of course, we try to react empathically, but it is almost impossible to share the feeling. Therefore, it is very important to include in therapy and research the subjective experiences of the clients and participants. We as music therapists and music therapy researchers should be as close as possible to the participants' experiences through "intimate knowledge." From this, it can be concluded that:

- Music therapy treatment should take place "in" experiences and should not be "about" experiences.
- The music therapist should join the client in his musical expression, not be an observer.
- Countertransference, which uses the personal experience of the music therapist to understand and describe the client's experience, is an adequate research tool.
- To understand deeply what happens in music therapy, you should be in the music therapy experience and not be just a spectator who looks at it from the outside.
- Researchers in music therapy should be modest, not claiming that they can know better the experiences of the client and music therapist. Researchers who make use of the symbolic type of knowledge should be aware that this knowledge is different from the intimate knowledge of the participants.
- Every effort to give music therapy referential meaning, by means of words, images, or figures, disregards the essence of music therapy.

This brings me to another question that again and again has been put forward: How can we discuss music therapy if words, images, and figures distract us from its essence? This is a tough question. In the sense of Steiner, I might answer: Do not write about music therapy, but join the session and experience the music therapy process yourself. Then you are in the essence of the experience, not in a secondary, deduced experience. However, stating that this is the only way to understand music therapy cannot satisfy. We need to translate music therapy into words, and take the risk that we reduce what it is all about: the client's and therapist's intra- and interpersonal experiences in sound.

Any time, we should be aware that words never can give us the experience of being in the music. When in Steiner's sense music is "irreducible," then the effort to describe music in words can give us only "empty" words. And as Wittgenstein (1999) wrote, we should keep silent and not talk about experiences that cannot be expressed in words. In Wittgenstein's opinion, a sentence of words only can tell us how it is, not what it is. By means of words, you can talk "about" it, but you cannot talk "it." In the next chapter, I will make a bridge from the nonreferential and nonsymbolic characteristics of music to a psychological and semiotic perspective that can explain why musical processes are analogous to psychological processes.

Chapter Five

ANALOGY: A CORE CATEGORY IN THE WRITINGS OF MUSIC THERAPISTS

INTRODUCTION

From Chapter Three, we can conclude that developing a "theory of music therapy" is an enterprise with several obstacles. From a qualitative point of view, theory is suspect. It makes no sense to proclaim universal laws when one tries to describe an ever-changing human context that gives rise to multiple subjective perspectives. And if someone wants to look at the many-sided human nature, it is impossible to reduce it to isolated variables. Therefore, some music therapists doubt the possibility of a general theory. However, even music therapists working with a qualitative paradigm adopt a theory—for instance, humanistic psychology—that is closely linked to the qualitative paradigm. Maybe it is not theory as such that is debatable, but what theory should look like.

The discussion about the possibility of a general theory of music therapy includes two other discussions. The first is centered on the topic of whether we should use a qualitative or a quantitative research paradigm. The second discussion, still going on, is about the question of whether music therapy should be connected to an already existing psychological theory of therapy, or instead should develop its own alternative theory.

Let me first explain my own perspective as a researcher. As a researcher, I am convinced that we need the qualitative paradigm and the quantitative paradigm as well. Because quantitative research is reductionistic, music therapists in this paradigm often miss what they feel belongs to the essence of music therapy. However, the discussion about research paradigms sometimes seems to become narrowed down to a normative one where qualitative research is glorified as "good," and quantitative research is labeled as "bad and ugly." In my view, both paradigms give answers to very different questions.

Maybe the intermediate position I advocate looks somehow like a paradox. If someone adopts the qualitative paradigm, how is it possible at another time to look through a quantitative pair of glasses? But, as in music listening, I believe and have experienced that it is possible at one time to listen to the "figure" and at another time to listen to the "ground" (or "essence") of human existence.

Concerning the discussion of whether we should develop our own theory or make connections with already existing theories, I say yes and no. I say yes, because we need a theory of music therapy that describes the analogy of musical and psychological processes in such a way that the essence and typical characteristics of music therapy are highlighted.

I say no, because we do not need our own theories of pathology and therapy. What we need is a theory of music therapy, not a theory of pathology and a theory of therapy. Music therapists should use the knowledge that has been gathered in other therapeutic professions. A music therapist working in psychiatry, for example, should be informed about diagnostic descriptions put forward by the American Psychiatric Association or the World Health Organization. Music therapists also should adopt knowledge about therapeutic processes that have been described in other therapeutic models. Of course, this cannot be the whole story, because if music therapists do not add knowledge, if they do not describe how disturbances and handicaps are expressed in music, if they are not able to describe musical processes that can cure disturbances and develop handicaps, then music therapy cannot be therapeutic.

Claiming a theory of music therapy does not mean refusing knowledge from other sources, but stresses the fact that music therapy can provide additional assessment data and therapeutic strategies. These data should be linked to already existing data from different sources. If not, the music therapist will be a Robinson Crusoe inventing his own very primitive tools.

In this chapter, I shall report the genesis of a theoretical perspective that can be part of a theory of music therapy. I do not claim to give a universal theory. I present one perspective, which first arose intuitively when I studied the work of my colleagues. At that time, I did not intend to develop a theory, and I did not have a pre-fixed qualitative research design to get there either.

At the start of my theoretical voyage of discovery, it was not clear at all that there could be a shared theoretical perspective. When I took off, I thought that music therapy should be divided along the lines of existing therapies, or disturbances and handicaps. However, gradually it became clear to me that in all those different perspectives there exists some shared idea about how music therapy works, and what is essential to music therapy.

First, I will go into some details of the qualitative research method, which I describe in retrospective. Next, I will describe the results of my research, especially the definition of the theoretical concept.

RESEARCH

In qualitative research, the researcher works without existing theories. He adopts no theory that gives him a priori statements. There are no prefixed concepts and no hypotheses by which relationships between concepts are proclaimed. No experiment is used to test hypotheses, and there are no measuring instruments to assess the values of the operationalized concepts.

The advantage of not using these procedures is that the naturalistic context is not distorted, and the descriptions of subjective experiences within this context are not reduced. The openness to the natural context makes it possible to develop new concepts that fit closely the natural context. Perhaps this fit is so close that generalization to other contexts is impossible.

The qualitative researcher does not believe there is an objective reality "out there," and is interested in subjective perspectives people develop to describe what they experience as their reality. Thus the qualitative researcher tries to find *constructed* meaning, and knows that constructed meaning is different from "truth."

The data I used are written-down descriptions and definitions music therapists themselves use when they communicate about music therapy. Music therapists are influenced by theories like humanistic psychology, psychoanalysis, morphology, behaviorism, and others, but to me it was a challenge to see whether, in spite of these different frameworks, there is some sort of a shared idea about music therapy.

There is one problem in doing this, because when concepts from different frameworks are put together, some aspects of the original meaning may be lost. However, something is won also when different concepts can become connected to each other.

The Core Category

When listening to music therapists, the listener is confronted with different concepts music therapists use to describe the music therapy processes. Concepts are verbal labels attached to the therapeutic phenomena to give them a name. Using a concept goes further than merely describing what is happening. Concepts are more abstract notions the concrete actions are subordinated to, such as, for instance, concepts such as "to assist," "to execute," and "to mediate." These concepts do not describe the concrete actions of a secretary. A concrete action, for example, is "taking notes." This action can be subordinated to the more abstract concept of "to assist."

Concepts can be grouped in categories. Strauss and Corbin (1990, p. 61) define a *category* as a classification that is discovered when concepts are compared and appear to belong to a similar phenomenon. Concepts are grouped together in a category, which itself is a more abstract concept. For instance, the concepts "to assist," "to execute," and "to mediate" can be part of the job description for "secretary." A *core* category is a central phenomenon around which several other categories can become integrated (Strauss & Corbin, 1990,

p. 116). Let me give you some *criteria* for a core category that I developed myself:

- Many music therapists should use the core category
- The core category acts as a metacategory, and thus should include other categories and have a central position between other categories
- Music therapists who use the core category should not belong to a single therapeutic school of music therapy
- The core category should be able to be applied to different disturbances and handicaps

Research Method

Doing qualitative research means working with an ever-developing design. When I give you the phases of research I went through, please realize that they developed spontaneously during the process of research.

The following research activities have been undertaken:

- Reading descriptions and definitions of music therapists communicating about their own work
- Identifying concepts that reflect the essential aspects in each individual's description
- Cross-analyzing and comparing the essential individual concepts of different music therapists
- Integrating these concepts into one category and signifying the category by means of a more abstract concept
- Using this category concept as a *sensitizing concept* when investigating new data
- Analyzing whether the category and the properties it signifies can fulfill the criteria of a core category
- Defining and redefining the properties of the core category

This chapter describes the research steps by which the core category has been developed. The final step, defining and redefining the core category, will be the topic of Chapter Seven. Chapter Six will be used to ground the core category in psychology and art theory.

EXAMPLES OF CONCEPTS USED BY MUSIC THERAPISTS

First, I'll give, in a chronological order, several examples of descriptions I found while exploring personal theories of music therapists:

- "The nature of the therapy session is best understood when thought of as *analogous* to a family or home situation" (Edith Hillman-Boxill, 1985, p. 23)
- "Improvisation is an *analogous* training space" (Gertrud Katja Loos, 1986, p. 162)
- "The building bricks of music (melody, sound, rhythm, dynamics, and form) are *analogies* of our way of thinking, feeling, and acting, and in our improvisations is expressed how we think, feel, and behave" (Isabelle Frohne-Hagemann, 1986, p. 18)
- "The multitude of sounding and rhythmic manifestations of music *corresponds* with the multitude of human existence in general" (Paulo Knill, 1987, p. 11)
- "For me there is no more clear *prototype* for the many paradoxes of the Gestalt development of the human soul as the phenomenon of a musical composition" (Rosemarie Tüpker, 1988, p. 48)
- "It may be inferred then that people become aware of the ground of their being not in verbal logic, but in a logic *analogous* to the ground of their own functioning (i.e., music)" (David Aldridge, 1989, p. 94)
- "Although the efforts take place within a musical framework, they are seen as a *metaphor* for what the client needs to learn or accomplish in life" (Ken Bruscia, 1989, p. 27)
- "The field of play is a space of experimentation, modeling, imitation in sound forms that express, *represent,* and communicate significant feelings, thoughts, attitudes, values, behavioral orientations, issues of growth and change" (Carolyn Kenny, 1989, p. 82)
- "The Nordoff-Robbins approach emphasizes the *congruence* between musical form and the Self" (David Aldridge, Gudrun Brandt, & Dagmar Wohler, 1990, p. 189)
- "There are *analogies* between the music therapeutic improvisation and the adaptation to body handicap" (Silke Jochims, 1990, p. 116)
- "The expressive features (of music), *correspond* with the dynamic forms of emotions" (Mercedes Pavlicevic, 1990, p. 6)
- "There was such a striking *concordance* between his musical

exploration and the quality of our relating" (Edith Lecourt, 1991, p. 93)

- "Music therapists hold the proposition that the musical expression of a patient and the musical interaction with the therapist *reflect* the central personality aspects of this patient" (Tonius Timmermann, Nicola Scheytt-Hölzer, Susanne Bauer, & Horst Kächele, 1991, p. 386)
- "The same way the fundamental values of mankind are founded on the category of temporarity (life/dead), so every musical composition in its temporarity is a precise *model* of human life" (Kimmo Lehtonen, 1994, p. 10)
- "This [the range of feelings expressed by group members] occurred primarily through the therapists' ability to improvise music that matched the feeling tone of individual group members' expressions, and this improvised, musical *analog* served both to convey the nature of the emotion that was communicated verbally and to compensate for what could not be expressed verbally" (Kenneth Aigen, 1995b, p. 350)
- "The components of music *touch* mental disturbances" (Fritz Hegi, 1997)
- "The processes of resonance and their misfits, which later on lead to psychopathology, are represented in a music therapy that is understood as psychotherapeutic, and are herein repeated" (Barbara Gindl, 2001)

There are a lot more of these descriptions (in music therapy and the other arts therapies as well), and I am sure that this short sample can give only a limited impression. But this limited impression is enough to demonstrate my point of view that music therapists share a central idea of how music therapy works.

From the music therapists' descriptions, basic concepts were deduced, which have been put in italics. Several music therapists use the concept of analogy. Other music therapists use concepts such as correspondence, prototype, metaphor, representation, congruence, concordance, reflection, model, and touch. In the next section, I tie all these concepts together in one category, which will be named "analogy."

ANALOGY AS A CORE CATEGORY

In a previous part, I gave four criteria for a category to be a core category. The first criterion (many music therapists should use the core category) has been illustrated with quotations in the previous section. Here, we will focus on the other three criteria and start with the criterion that a core category should include other categories and have a central position between other categories.

When different concepts are put into one category and subordinated under one central abstract concept, we must ask ourselves if these different concepts indeed "... appear to belong to a similar phenomenon" (Strauss & Corbin, 1990, p. 61), and what the central concept of this category of concepts should be.

All quotations in the previous section and the concepts that have been deduced from them signify somehow the link between the musical processes and the intra- and interpersonal processes. Some of them state more explicitly that the context of music therapy is a playspace where a client in the context of musical activities can explore intra- and interpersonal processes.

Because of these two reasons, in my opinion the quotations belong to a similar phenomenon and can be put into one category. I haven chosen the concept of analogy as the central concept to signify this category because in the quotations "analogy" is used by several music therapists, and because it is used also in Stern's developmental psychology that is of great help in constituting the link between the musical processes and the intra- and interpersonal processes (which I will define as the link between the forms of perception and the forms of feeling; see next chapter).

Now let us focus on the important question of why analogy should be a *core* category in the theory of music therapy. There are several reasons to nominate analogy as a core category.

First, because "analogy" implies "same and different": There is a context in which actions are different from outside life reality but the experiences that are evoked by these actions are real. "Same and different" is basic to what happens during music therapy.

Second, it can take a central position between other categories to which it can be linked. To illustrate the last argument, take one example. The concept of *creativity*, which itself signifies a category, is less central than analogy. Maybe to music therapists who call themselves creative music therapists this looks strange. In a general view, of course, they are right, because in music therapy the client and the music therapist *create* music, and thereby "...develop and expand both their own (the therapist's) and their clients' responses" (Forinash, 1992, p. 130). This definition makes every therapy a creative therapy.

However, if we want to use a more focused description of "creativity" and take a view that is based on client-centered indications and rationales, our thoughts will be different. Then the creative process can be described as one type of a process that enables the client to become more creative, which means that he frees himself from fixed ideas, behaviors, and feelings. This creative process can be indicated with particular types of neurotic disturbances, but cannot be used anytime, anywhere, anyhow. Take, for example, the treatment of clients with early childhood disturbances that need to be expressed and worked through. Is it appropriate to take changing fixed ideas, behaviors, and feelings as treatment goals? To give expression to what is suppressed seems to be a more appropriate goal. Concepts such as expression, transference, empathy, symbolization, structuring, and others are reflected incompletely in the category of creativity. This explains why not every music therapist wants to call himself a creative therapist.

If one looks at treatment modalities such as supportive, palliative, developmental, re-educative, and reconstructive, and their methodical implications (see Chapter Two), it becomes clear that the creative process in a more focused definition cannot be the appropriate method for all these different treatment modalities. Therefore, the category of creativity cannot be a core category of music therapy. Concepts such as creativity, expression, transference, empathy, symbolization, structuring, and others all are categories. Let me give you several examples to illustrate that these categories can be subsumed under the core category of analogy.

In *transference,* the client experiences the relationship to the therapist as a relationship stemming from previous experiences. The client projects characteristics of a significant person in his life on the therapist and experiences the therapist as being that person. The client perhaps expects or claims the therapist to behave as the significant person. Let us suppose that the therapist is experienced as a nurturing mother. In music therapy, this process of transference comes to birth in music. Nurturance is possible because the musical interaction is similar to the very first mother-child interaction. In other words, the musical process is an analogy of the early mother-child interaction. One also could say that because an important part of the mother-child interaction in essence is musical (see next chapter).

Symbolization in music therapy often is made possible because of analogy. Symbolization means that something refers to something else. In music therapy, musical instruments, musical parameters, and musical processes can have symbolic meaning. For instance, playing on a conga can represent a parent who is upset and reacts angrily to a child's behavior. In this case, this symbolization is made possible because there is analogy between the musical form and characteristics of the parent's behavior.

Take another example (taken from Tüpker, 1988/1996). A musical improvisation that is made up of broken-off parts that are unconnected with each other symbolized the childhood of a child raised in an orphanage without continuous care and holding. As an adult, the client's musical form symbolizes his discontinuous life development. The musical form can symbolize this life development because of the analogy between musical form and psychological development in time. The temporal forms of both phenomena (music and psychological development) are alike.

Symbolization can happen by analogous processes, but it can also happen merely by a process of association without analogy. Then there is no resemblance between the music process and its meaning. However, symbolization in itself cannot be a core category, because it is used only in particular treatments.

Distinct psychological schools of music therapy—the humanistic, the psychoanalytic, the morphologic, the Gestalt, the behavioral, and others—each describe important psychological processes and musical processes that can be used in treatment. They all represent important perspectives on the human being, on therapy, and on music therapy more particularly. But none of these concepts can claim supremacy. What has been said about creativity, then, should be said about transference and symbolization, too. Transference and symbolization can be put into music, but both concepts are not universal to music therapy, which means that they are not part of most methods and treatments of music therapy. If there is no transference or symbolization, there still is analogy, when musical action in music therapy sounds the intra- and interpersonal process.

Two other criteria I put forward were that music therapists who use the core category should not belong to a single therapeutic school of music therapy, and that the core category should be able to be applied to different disturbances and handicaps.

The quotations I gave are from music therapists with divergent views: from Gestalt therapy, integrative therapy, psychoanalysis, expressive therapy, morphological psychology, humanistic psychology, developmental psychology, and anthroposophy. The quotations also are representative of working with the developmentally disabled, the autistic, the bodily handicapped, and the mentally disturbed.

I do not want to play down these differences. I think that these differences can be very fruitful. What I am saying is that in spite of these differences, there seems to be a shared fundamental understanding about music therapy. Some of the music therapists use the concept of analogy explicitly, whereas others use it more implicitly.

Finally, I want to mention that I am not claiming that this core category can be used in every context, or can subsume every music therapy process. Nevertheless, in my opinion it signifies one of the important core categories of music therapy.

EPILOGUE: TRIANGULATION

It has been shown that many music therapists share the idea that the client's thoughts, feelings, and behaviors are sounded in musical processes. As we shall see in the next chapter, this is the case because musical processes and psychological processes are composed of the same basic (amodal) parameters. The same holds true for processes of change and development. Because musical processes sound the basic parameters of psychological processes, music therapy is possible. This sounding of intra- and interpersonal processes in music has been conceptualized in the core category of "analogy."

Future research is needed to compare the psychological processes of mental disturbances and handicaps, and the processes of curing and development with musical processes. Music therapists from different roots, working with different client groups, should describe the musical processes used by them in an intermediary language that links the parameters of music to the parameters of the psyche.

What we need is a worldwide exchange and discussion by clinical experts. We need a triangulation of research methods; of sources; of clinical methods, rationales, and theoretical perspectives. Perhaps then it will be possible to generate a theoretical overview of music therapy in which core categories and categories are described that are differentiated but also integrated, so that we can offer our clients the best music therapy treatment there is, and successfully explain to everybody who wants to know just why and how music therapy works.

Chapter Six

FORMS OF FEELING AND FORMS OF PERCEPTION[6]

INTRODUCTION

When I started developing concepts for a general theory of music therapy, I originally used the words "sound" and "sound progression" to illustrate that in music therapy it is not music as a cultural/artistic phenomenon (the music of the concert hall) that is relevant, but sounds and sound progressions as expressions of the client's psyche. I defined "sound" to include all musical parameters: rhythm, dynamics, melody, harmony, timbre, and so on.

However, I gave it a second thought and decided not to continue using the words "sound" and "sound progression," because these words can easily be misinterpreted as methods of sound therapy and sound healing, which in my view lack the therapeutic relationship.

What is more, in the discussion with my colleagues it became clear to me that for music therapists the statement that music in music therapy does not refer to the cultural/artistic phenomenon is controversial. Such a statement seems to exclude the methods of receptive music therapy and seems to exclude the possibility that the well-formed can be therapeutic.

What I intended to say, when making the statement that in music therapy it is not music as a cultural/artistic phenomenon that is relevant, was that in music therapy the essence of music is the psychological process it sounds.[7] In other words, not the well-formed as such is healing, but the correspondence of the formed musical process and the psychological process of change of the client. This can be a well-formed musical process or not. I do not believe that the mere aesthetic experience of the well-formed in itself is healing if the musical form does not sound the inner processes and psychological changes of the client. Still, because my statement seems to obscure my intention, I decided to keep using the word "music."

---

[6]This chapter has been published also in the *Nordic Journal of Music Therapy* (2003) in the series "Theory Building in Music Therapy--An International Archive." Parts of it have been presented during conferences and were prepared in earlier publications.

[7]As said before, I use the word "sounding" instead of "reflecting."

In this chapter, I will ground the core category of analogy in psychology and art theory. I will discuss two perspectives, one taken from psychology and one from art, which can be of help to construct the connection between the musical and the psychological, between the arrangement of musical elements and the psychological meaning of these arrangements.

TO BEGIN WITH: THE HYPOTHESIS AND ONE EXAMPLE

Hypothesis

The fundamental characteristic of music therapy in my opinion is that playing, singing, and listening to music "sounds" the inner psyche of the client who plays, sings, and listens. In music therapy, the client expresses his psyche in music. The music therapist meets the client in his music.

Basic to music therapy theory is the concept that there is a correspondence between intra- and interpersonal experiences and expressions in music, and that there is a mutual correspondence between daily life experiences and expressions in music.

Example

Let me first give an example of these correspondences. Say that a person has a need to overcompensate his feelings of inferiority (intrapsychological). This need will affect his behavioral expressions when fulfilling his job tasks, when communicating with other people, and when expressing himself in activities such as improvising in music. When fulfilling his job tasks, he might force himself to be engaged in problems that are difficult to tackle. During communication, he might put himself into a very dominant position, talking with a loud voice, in a high speed, without rests, interrupting others. Driving his car from home to work can be fast and agitated. Improvising on musical instruments can be impulsive, complex, loud, and fast.

The expressions in different modes of behavior are not exactly identical. There is no linear correspondence between the inner experience and the outer expression, or between all outer expressions. However, in many cases there will be some expressions that correspond with the inner psyche and with other expressions. Because there are no linear correspondences between inner experiences and outer expressions, a therapist needs to focus on the individual expressions of each client, to find out. If he observes the client carefully, he will find characteristic expressions from which he can infer the client's inner experiences. And, of course, he should help the client to understand the match between inner experiences and outer expressions.

A PERSPECTIVE FROM PSYCHOLOGY

Introduction

The arts therapies should develop theories that are art-based. Nevertheless, these theories should be supported by evidence from psychology and therapy, because the arts therapies are meant to cure psychological diseases and handicaps. In this section, I'll focus on this supportive evidence from psychology. More particularly, I'll focus on evidence that is able to explain the correspondence between a person's inner experiences and his expressions in music.

One of the most important theories for music therapists is the developmental psychology of Stern (1985, 1995). It is important because it is music-based, and thus is able to secure the essential characteristics of music therapy. In this part, I want to elaborate on perception and vitality affects and show that the equality of the amodal characteristics of vitality affects and the musical parameters can explain the connection between the musical expression and the person's intra- and interpersonal processes.

Stern's concepts of amodal perception and vitality affects give us a perspective from developmental psychology that shows that the musical is the psychological and vice versa.

Cross-modal and Amodal Perception

Cross-modal perception refers to the possibility to perceive qualities (properties) that belong to one modality of perception (for instance, vision) in another modality of perception (for example, hearing). There are several examples of these cross-modal transpositions.

- *Cross-modality of physical form between the tactile and the visual modality.* It has been proved by Meltzoff and Borton (1979) that when the baby has a nipple in his mouth (tactile modality) before seeing it, he recognizes the physical form of the nipple when it is shown to him afterwards (visual modality).
- *Cross-modality of intensity between the auditory and the visual modality.* A correspondence between the auditory modality and the visual modality is possible when in both modalities intensity is

concerned (Lewcowics & Turkewitz, 1980). If a flash of lightning has the same intensity form as a sound that previously has been heard, then the baby will be able to recognize the correspondence between sound and light.

- *Cross-modality of temporal form between the auditory and the visual modality.* Lewcowics (1992) showed that babies could recognize the correspondence between a temporal form in the auditory modality when it is presented in the visual modality. The rhythm of a sound is experienced as equal to the same rhythm of a flash of light.

From the fact that babies are able to transpose a form from one modality to another, that they are able to recognize the visual analogy of a tactile form, the visual analogy of an auditory form, and vice versa, Stern concludes that they are able to represent tactile, visual, and auditory forms without words and symbols. The transposition from one modality to another modality is possible because the baby has an abstract amodal representation of the physical form, intensity, and temporal form, which acts as an intermediary bridge from one to another modality.

Important for the theory of analogy, which is the topic of this book, is that Stern states that the infant's experiences are beyond words and symbols. Concerning early parent-infant interactions, Stern tells us: "The actions do not symbolize anything. They are what it is about" (1995, p. 64).

Also important is that there exist amodal representations that can be recognized in any perceptual modality, and, as we shall see in the next section, that there exist "analogies" between the forms of perception and the forms of feeling, and that the parameters that make these analogies possible are art-based.

Vitality Affects

Until now, we have focused on cross-modality, the transposition between modalities of perception, which is made possible by amodal representations. However, in the interaction between the mother and the baby, and also in therapy, the most important transposition takes place from *feeling* to *perception* and vice versa. In music therapy, there is a transposition from feeling to perception in the music. How can forms of perception be transposed into forms of feeling and vice versa? Let us go back where it all starts, the nonverbal and nonsymbolic communication of the baby and its mother.

When a baby experiences joy (form of feeling), he will express this joy in a smile on his face (visual modality). The mother then can answer by smiling too (same modality). What Stern found out is that mothers are used to answer in different modalities. For instance, they make a sound (auditory modality) that lasts as long as the smile and goes up and down like the baby's lips and cheeks.

The baby "understands" that the mother's sound is an empathic answer to his smile and thus his joy. Stern tells us that it is this cross-modality and not the imitation in the same modality that communicates empathy to the baby. Essential to this example is the fact that an inner experience, the feeling of joy, corresponds with a perceptual form (smiling), which then is transposed to the auditory modality (sounds) to communicate empathy.

According to Stern (1985, p. 56), the infant experiences this as empathy, not knowing the denotative meaning of his mother's behavior. The baby does not interpret the mother's behavior. Sterns describes the communication of mother and baby as an abstract dance or piece of music. They are not "talking about" something else by means of verbal symbols, nor making gestures that refer to persons, things, or happenings. Thus there is no external "meaning."

Some time ago, Meyer (1970) introduced the concept of "embodied meaning," which is nonreferential, to illustrate that musical form is equal to psychological meaning, without the need for symbolization. He used Gestalt laws such as "closing" and "good continuation," which lead to some sort of "emotion" when they are disturbed. What Meyer proposed was a link between psychological processes (the Gestalt laws) and the experience of these laws in music. In other words, music is meaningful not because it represents something outside itself, but because musical processes in itself are psychological processes.

With Stern's concepts of cross-modality, amodality, and vitality affects, a similar line of reasoning is possible that links perception to feeling. Meyer's perspective from Gestalt psychology, where Gestalt laws evoke emotions, is limited because these emotions cannot cover all forms of feeling. Stern's connection of forms of feeling to perceptual forms is much more useful. Instead of "embodied meaning," he offers us "acts of meaning: events that are directly perceived and apprehended right away in terms of meanings" (Stern, 1995, p. 89).

Now let us go deeper into the forms of feeling as described by Stern. Stern defines *vitality affects* as the dynamic, kinetic qualities of feeling, such as "surging," "fading away," "fleeting," "explosive," "crescendo," "decrescendo," "bursting," and "drawn out," which should be distinguished from categorical affects such as being happy, sad, or angry (Stern, 1985, p. 54).

Because musical terms such as crescendo and decrescendo are used, this definition shows immediately that there is a close connection between perceptual forms and forms of feeling. Stern puts forward that "dance and music are examples par excellence of the expressiveness of vitality affects" (Stern, 1985, p. 56). Research on vitality affects and the arts therapies shows that the concept of vitality affect can be used for all arts therapies (see Smeijsters, 2000/2003). This makes it clear that Stern's developmental psychology is art-based.

When it is possible to describe music with the same dynamic kinetic terms as "surging, fading away, fleeting, explosive, crescendo, decrescendo, bursting, drawn out, and so on," which have been used by Stern when describing vitality affects, then we may conclude that this explains why there is an analogy between musical and psychological processes. When it is possible to describe the musical and psychological processes by means of the same dynamic terms, the analogies between musical forms and forms of feeling are apparent. The definition shows also which musical forms and which forms of feeling are analogous to each other (for other arts therapies, this can be different).

As Stern points out, vitality affects can be there in the presence or absence of categorical affects: "... a 'rush' of anger or of joy, a perceived flooding of light, an accelerating sequence of thoughts, an unmeasurable wave of feeling evoked by music, and a shot of narcotics can all feel like 'rushes' ..." (Stern, p. 55). What is common in these phenomena is the way in which the process of the phenomenon unfolds as a pattern in time and intensity.

It is not the referring signal or symbol, which signifies categorical feelings, that counts, but the "way of feeling" that is expressed in a pattern in time and intensity. What is more, these patterns in time and intensity are everywhere; they are psychological as well as nonpsychological. This makes it possible to grasp the sameness of time and intensity patterns in different types of processes and different modalities of expression. For example, you can experience a form of feeling in the dynamics of weather conditions.

Because a person is able to perceive these patterns in different processes and modalities of expression, it is possible to express and perceive intra- and interpersonal forms of feeling in patterns of music. We can express ourselves and understand each other's feelings by the transmutation of forms of feeling into musical forms of perception, and by the retransmutation of the musical forms of perception back into forms of feeling (Stern, 1985, p. 159). Thus, the forms of music are similar to the basic forms of the subjective, nonverbal intra- and interpersonal experiences. In the musical and the psychological process, there is a similar unfolding of time and intensity.

Stern calls the *protonarrative envelopes* the building blocks of each person's implicit relational knowing. With the concept of the protonarrative envelope, he describes the "dramatic line of tension [that] is invariably synchronous with the temporal feeling shape [as it emerges during the present moment]" (Stern, 1995, p. 91). It is called "proto" because it is a preverbal narrative.

It is important, as Stern et al. (1998) point out, that the implicit relational knowing is not unique to the presymbolic infant but continues throughout life. From childhood until old age, in all our encounters with other people the dramatic lines of tension, the feeling shapes, give us important implicit personal knowing. This implicit personal knowing can make us healthy when there is attunement, but it can make us sick when there is misattunement. The clinically important moments are those moments of meeting that rearrange the implicit relational knowing. Then there is a sudden qualitative change in relationship. Therapists are there to make it possible that misattunement can be cured and implicit relational knowing can change. It is in music therapy that the protonarrative envelopes of the implicit relational knowing become expressed in sound and can be turned into healthy envelopes.

Because during lifetime the implicit relational knowing is always there, everyone—parents, partners, friends, colleagues, bosses—should take care that misattunement is prevented.

Examples From Music Therapy

In this section, I will give a short overview to illustrate what has been said before (extended examples will be given in Chapter Nine).

Imagine a music therapist who adjusts his music to the face expressions and movements of his client. There are many situations in music therapy (for instance, when working with the mentally handicapped or the autistic) when a music therapist is operating like this. When a client is producing vocal or instrumental sounds himself, then the music therapist attunes to the client's sounds. What is different from Stern's examples is that the music therapist is answering in the same modality. By doing this, music therapist and client share the client's personal world in an intermediary "space" (Kenny, 1989) of music. Although music therapist and client are expressing themselves in the same modality, there is the transposition from forms of feeling into forms of perception. Let me explain this further.

What the music therapist and the client are doing when improvising in active music therapy is not just "playing music." Music therapy improvisation is not improvising as in jazz, pop/rock, or classical improvisation. Jazz, pop/rock, and classical improvisers are playing around with musical motifs with the aim of spontaneously constructing musical forms that make "musical sense." Introducing a motif, which rhythmically is varied, accelerated, varied in contour, ornamented, played in another key, supported by variations of harmonics, and so on—in other words, developing an improvisation along the musical lines of jazz, pop/rock, or classical improvisation—is not the aim of music therapy. Jazz, pop/rock, and classical improvisations are pushed forward by aesthetic rules. Music therapy is not an aesthetic affair. In music therapy, it is not "aesthetic form" but "psychological form" that counts. The same holds true for receptive music therapy and more art-based forms of active music therapy (playing and singing composed tunes and so on).

Thus, what is essential for music therapy is that it is a "psychological affair." The musical processes in the intermediary musical space are experienced and interpreted as expressions of the psyche. Neither "musical" ability nor aptitude is assessed, nor is it developed. In music therapy, the client in the music sounds his Self, how he behaves, how he feels, and how he expresses his conflicts. The "aesthetic" meaning is unimportant; it does not matter whether it sounds like an artistic form. What is important is that the music sounds as the client's psyche.

The musical improvisation offers the client an opportunity to express his Self in musical form. This does not mean that precomposed pieces of music, which for example are used in Guided Imagery and Music, and precomposed traditional tunes in active music therapy have less value. In musical improvisation and in working with precomposed music, it is the form of feeling that is sounded in the "perceptual form" of the music that counts. And, of course, the music can evoke purely aesthetic experiences, it can have associations, it can have symbolic meaning, it can be linked to words, and so on. All these things are part of music therapy. However, the essence of music therapy is the match between the perceptual forms of music and the forms of feeling.

In the past, several theories of music therapy claimed that listening to or playing musical pieces and singing songs will improve health. I am not countering this completely, but in my opinion this can only be the case if the perceptual forms of these songs and pieces of music are expressions of the clients' forms of feeling. If they are not, listening to pieces of music is just a matter of preference, which is a "psychological" issue of course, but does not change the client's Self. The aim of music therapy is a change of the client's forms of feeling by means of changing his musical forms. Not the music as such, but the forms of feeling, which they sound, is the focus. The music therapist supports the client in putting his Self into music, and in exploring possible changes of the Self in the music. It is the premise of music therapy that a client changes when his music changes. If an improvisation offers the client the possibility to express himself in music, then a change in music signifies a personal change. Learning to improvise along classical, pop/rock, or jazz guidelines enhances the improvisational abilities and perhaps enhances the general learning ability; it does not change the deeper areas of the psyche.

Changes in the ability for jazz, pop/rock, and classical improvisation and changes in musical preferences are not indicative of deeper personal changes (in pop/rock improvisation, for instance, with its roots in blues, this is different, because in this case a solo is led by a form of feeling, which is psychological, not musical). Deeper personal changes will occur only when changes do not result from a change in musical technique or preference, but from a change in music that sounds the inner psyche.

Now let us look at some examples from clients that show how forms of feeling are expressed in forms of music, and how forms of feeling can be changed by changes in musical forms.

When a severely depressive person expresses himself by playing in a very slow tempo and soft dynamics, this musical expression may reflect his inner state of mind. I write "may" because there are no universal linear connections between the forms of feeling and the musical forms. Each client is a unique person who expresses himself in a unique way. Nevertheless, research has showed that there are equivalences between the characteristics of disturbances and the expression in music. When a client comes into music therapy, he takes his thoughts, feelings, and behaviors with him, which he expresses in music in a unique way, but they are still characterized by his disturbance. The music therapist can offer changes in tempo, rhythm, and dynamics to give an opportunity to the client to transform into another way of being.

When a compulsive client repeats the same rhythm or melody all the time, the behavior in music sounds his compulsion. The music therapist can help him to accept and imitate slight changes in rhythm or melody, and help him to accept and imitate an alternation between the stereotyped motif and a new motif introduced by the music therapist.

In both examples, the music expresses the inner being of the client. Changes in the music reflect personal changes. One might object that it is possible to describe these examples by musical techniques of composition. In the first case of depression, the music therapist introduces an accelerando and crescendo; in the second case of compulsion, the music therapist introduces variation and an alternating structure (A-B-A). However, the musical focus of the music therapist differs from the focus of a musician. The music therapist is not a music teacher who teaches accelerandi, crescendi, variations, and musical structures. The music therapist in the music hears the psyche of the client, and introduces changes in the music because of their psychological significance.

Just as the verbal therapist is talking to someone about his feelings, the music therapist "talks" by means of music. He listens, shows empathy through music, and through music offers possibilities for how to change the client's feelings, and to let him set foot on other areas of experience. The music therapist operates musical techniques that result in musical processes that reflect personal changes. The music therapist does not have the musical techniques in his mind. In his mind is the "person as music" and the change of the "person in music."

Let me give some additional examples. From quantitative research, we know that playing slow can be an analogy of manifest depressive behavior (Steinberg, 1987; Steinberg & Raith, 1985).

Jochims (1990) and Heal (1991) described the analogy between the psychological process a client undergoes after a traffic accident that made him handicapped, and taking part in a musical improvisation. The client, who suddenly becomes severely handicapped, has to change his life, his plans, and his activities. In an instant, he has to say farewell to his previous life. In a free musical improvisation, one has to be flexible and to develop the ability to adjust one's musical behavior immediately to the suddenly changing musical surrounding. One tries to predict the musical process, but suddenly it can change completely. This can be frustrating, because what one was developing musically is suddenly stopped. Like the life situation after an accident, the musical improvisation frustrates and requests frustration tolerance, coping behavior, and the ability to be flexible and to adjust. The way a client behaves in the musical improvisation sounds if he is able to adjust himself to the new situation. By means of music therapy, the client can learn to adjust to sudden changes and to tolerate frustration. Of course, such an analogy between the urge for changing your life and the constant adjustment to the changes in the musical improvisation should be recognized by the client and worked through. But what is important is that the client in his musical process experiences the forms of feeling he experiences in normal life when coping with his handicap.

Results of my own qualitative single-case studies show that playing a fixed pattern of rhythm can be analogous to compulsive behavior (Van den Hurk & Smeijsters, 1991), and the alternating of a fast melodic line with a robust melodic motif turned out to be an expression of bad communication between a client and her mother (Smeijsters & Van den Hurk, 1993). Sounds arising suddenly, with an outburst of dynamics, with a rude timbre, and with colliding harmonics have been described by a client as an analogy of being hit (Smeijsters & Van den Berk, 1995/1999). Playing loud, not willing to adjust to someone else's musical grounding, turned out to be an analogy of a child taking over the leading role from her mother, not wanting to obey (Smeijsters & Storm, 1997/1998). Not being able to find a free melodic line has been described as an expression analogous to a lack of personal identity (Smeijsters & Van den Hurk, 1999).

Nowadays in music therapy publications, references to Stern's developmental psychology are very frequent (for example, Bunt, 1994; Aldridge, 1996; Pavlicevic, 1997; Hegi, 1997, 1998; Schumacher, 1994, 1999, and many others). Hegi makes a connection between musical parameters and early childhood experiences as described by Stern. He sees a resemblance between the ways Stern observes babies and the ways music therapists decode nonverbal musical expressions. The person, Hegi says, "talks" in the music, and by means of "trans-sensorial" analogies, a bridge is established from music to inner presentations. Schumacher used Stern's work in her research on autistic clients.

Hegi and Schumacher both make a connection between Stern's phases of development and musical experiences. Table 6.1 gives a summary of Schumacher's indications for music therapy, which she describes along the developmental phases of Stern.

Table 6.1

*Indications for Music Therapy Based on Stern's Developmental Phases**

Prenatal Self

- Disturbances: preterm babies, coma patients
- Aims: decreasing isolation, experiencing interpersonal contact, maintaining the mother-child relationship
- Music therapy: by means of music making contact to the outer world

Emergent Self

- Disturbances: perceptual disturbances caused by a lack of intermodal integration,** autism, psychosis, borderline personality disorder
- Aims: integration of sensory perception
- Music therapy: music as a multisensorial stimulus stimulates intermodal integration

Core Self

- Disturbances: disturbance of body awareness, Rett syndrome, neurological disturbances, early disturbances such as eating disorders and borderline personality disorder
- Aims: experiencing body awareness, self-agency, self-coherence, self-history, self-affectivity, time flow
- Music therapy: music compensates the lack of body awareness, music makes it possible to work through the lack of affect attunement, music can communicate early traumatic conflicts

Subjective Self

- Disturbances: not being able to share feelings with another person, psychosomatic disturbances, disturbances of attachment
- Aims: perceiving yourself and the others correctly, balancing nearness/distance, making contact effectively, working through psychological conflicts, symbolizing and verbalizing
- Music therapy: music doubles the Self and makes it possible to listen to yourself and to be listened to by others

*Based on Schumacher, 1999, pp. 92–95.

**Intermodal integration means that a person is able to perceive the same amodal patterns in different stimuli. It makes reality much easier to understand.

Concerning Table 6.1, more worldwide research is needed to make sure that the content within the cells and the connections between the cells are valid. For instance, the hypothesis that autism, psychosis, and the borderline personality all can be described as a lack of intermodal integration should be grounded in tough empirical evidence. In my opinion, the lack of intermodal integration indeed is part of the syndromes, but leaves information out about understanding the syndrome's typical characteristics and its appropriate specified treatment.

Schumacher did very important work in the research on autism, where she links Stern's developmental phases to autism, to its expression in music, to appropriate music therapy goals and techniques (her findings will be included in Table 6.2 also). She makes it very clear that vitality affects and attunement are based on musical parameters such as rhythm, tempo, meter, intensity, and melodic contour. Schumacher developed an assessment scale, which makes it possible to assess the levels of attunement in the musical interaction. This kind of research should be continued for other disturbances as well.

Table 6.2 gives a more detailed description of Stern's developmental phases and how they can be used in music therapy; Hegi's and Schumacher's findings are included.

Table 6.2

Stern's Developmental Stages and Equivalent Experiences in Music

Developmental Phases of the Emergent Self

- Cross-modal Perception

  Definition: to take information received in one sensory modality and somehow translate it into another sensory modality (disturbances: learning disabilities)*

  Experience in music: music therapist transposes the client's behavioral patterns into sound, transposes all kind of sensory patterns into sound, and vice versa
- The Perception of Vitality Affects

  Definition: dynamic shifts or patterned changes within ourselves (disturbances: anxiety disorders)

  Experience in music: music therapist sounds the client's behavioral expressions of vitality affects

Developmental Phases of the Core Self (starts at age 2–3 months)

- Self-agency

  Definition: the sense of authorship of one's own actions; the sense of volition that precedes a motor act, having control over

self-generated action, and predictability of consequences that follow the act (disturbances: psychosis, catatonia, hysterical paralysis, derealization, paranoid states)
Experience in music: the client explores the effects of actions on musical instruments, takes control and changes musical motifs, initiates new musical motifs, influences the musical play of the music therapist and other clients

- Self-coherence
  Definition: having a sense of being a nonfragmented, physical whole with boundaries, and a locus of integrated action. It includes the experience that something is in one place at one time (unity of locus), that things that move coherently in time belong together (coherence of motion), that many behaviors that are invariably performed simultaneously by one person share a common temporal structure (coherence of temporal structure), that behaviors that are performed together share a common intensity structure (coherence of intensity structure), that someone else has a form that belongs to him (coherence of form) (disturbances: psychosis, depersonalization, fragmentation, merger or fusion)
  Experience in music: the client produces musical sounds in a coherent way, with integrated movements; experiences his musical playing as acting in the here-and-now in one place and at one time; experiences his musical play as a whole, with a temporal structure, intensity, and form; experiences the musical play of others as a whole, with a temporal structure and intensity
- Self-affectivity
  Definition: experiencing patterned inner qualities of feeling (affects) that belong with other experiences of Self (proprioceptive feedback, internally patterned sensations of arousal or activation, emotion-specific qualities of feeling) (disturbances: psychosis, anhedonia)
  Experience in music: the client experiences forms of music as forms of feeling, belonging to one's Self
- Self-history
  Definition: having the sense of enduring, of a continuity with one's past so that one "goes on being" and can even change while remaining the same (disturbances: psychosis, fugue, dissociation)
  Experience in music: the client experiences himself as a musical form with a past, a present, and a future, with motifs

that change and motifs that are repeated, a mix of same and different that belongs to him

- Self-regulating Other

  Definition: there is someone who regulates the self-experiences of the infant (the arousal, affect intensity, security and attachment)

  Experience in music: the music therapist contains the client's exploration of musical forms, and introduces conservation and variation of form parts

- Self-regulating Experiences with Things

  Definition: the personification of things, which are able to evoke and regulate feelings of the infant

  Experience in music: the client develops musical motifs that become transitional objects

Developmental Phases of the Subjective Self (starts at the seventh month). The child knows that others have subjective experiences that can be shared (disturbances: pervasive feeling of aloneness, anxiety for intimacy, false Self, splitting, neurotic symptoms such as displacement, personality disorders).

- Sharing the Focus of Attention

  Definition: the gesture of pointing and the act of following one another's lines of vision

  Experience in music: the music therapist and the clients attend and develop together musical form

- Sharing Intentions

  Definition: acts directed at a referent person (such as reaching out a hand to get a cookie), which imply that the infant attributes an internal mental state to that person

  Experience in music: the music therapist and the clients dialogue in the music, make spaces, and invite the co-player to have an input that fits the previous musical form. See Bruscia (1987).**

- Sharing Affective States

  Definition: to look toward the mother to read her face for its affective content, which tells the infant how he should feel in situations of uncertainty. The infant attributes to the mother the capacity of having a signal and affect that has relevance to his own actual or potential feeling states.

  Experience in music: the music therapist and the clients share the feeling states that are expressed in the music

- Affect Attunement

  Definition: The cross-modal matching of some aspect of the behavior that reflects a person's feeling state. The match refers not to the external behavior, but to the expression of an inner state. It is behavior as expression, not as a sign or symbol. The vehicles of transfer are metaphor and analogy. The match is made by intensity, tempo, rhythm, duration, and form.

Experience in music: the music therapist and the clients, by means of musical forms, match one another's inner feeling state, and understand one another's musical behaviors as forms of feeling. The music therapist uses techniques such as pacing and reflecting, by which he does not imitate, but instead matches the energy level (intensity, speed) and feelings exhibited by the client. See Bruscia (1987).

Developmental Phases of the Verbal Self (starts at the second year). The child is able to tell a story about his life. There is a distance between the lived experience and the verbal representation

- An Objective View of the Self

  Definition: the child knows that he can be objectified, represented in some form that exists outside of his subjectively felt Selves

  Experience in music: the client experiences himself sounded in a musical product

- Symbolic Play

  Definition: the child is able by means of toys to represent situations

  Experience in Music: the client sounds persons and events by means of musical play. The music therapist uses techniques such as symbolizing, which makes an instrument or a musical motif to represent a person or an event. See Bruscia (1987).

- The Use of Language

  Definition: by means of a verbal dialogue, a new way of relating is possible. The child is able to tell his own life story (disturbances: rationalization, repression, denial)

*Disturbances and disabilities that lack the particular abilities are included.
**This table gives only some examples of Bruscia's techniques that can be used.

Concerning Table 6.2, much more research is needed to validate the match between Stern's developmental phases and the client's experiences in music therapy. (For art therapists, the work of Rutten-Saris is important. She researched Stern's developmental phases for art therapy. See the references.)

Conclusion of the Psychological Perspective

Fundamental to the theory of analogy is that musical processes sound psychological processes, and that music therapy enables the client to change his vitality affects by means of changing his forms of music. A depressive client can experience new vitality affects by means of accelerandi and crescendi. A compulsive client, by means of variations, can loosen his stereotyped rhythms and melodic fragments.

The music therapist is the one who hears the musical process as a psychological process and makes arrangements to transform psychological processes in musical processes. He listens to the client's music, reacts by means of musical attunement, and offers musical possibilities who make possible changes in the client's vitality affects.

Musical processes are supported by talks in which the analog experiences of the clients are verbalized. This talk can take place through a phenomenological description of what happened in the psyche in the music, or by a hermeneutical interpretation, which gives symbolic meaning to the musical event. However, the essence of the music therapy lies in the experience of the form of feeling as it appears in the present forms of music.

When identifying the psychological process and the musical process too absolutely, it looks as if music as such is therapeutic. However, music as an aesthetic structure has its own rules, and not every musical rule has psychological significance. If a client's music-making improves, this automatically does not mean that he is cured. For example, when a client changes his random playing into an A-B-A structure, of course this is an aesthetic improvement, but to be sure that it is a psychological improvement, we need to ask which psychological process is sounded in this musical change.

I am not convinced that making music is therapeutic in itself anyway. I would like to have a close look into the musical processes and describe what a person is experiencing when the musical process unfolds. I think that we need to define musical processes as psychological processes and decide which musical process should be used according to the client's psychological needs. Contrary to the statement that "music therapists are artists," I would say this: "Music therapists are therapists who act like artists." Music therapists are not musicians who listen to and follow the rules of music; they are therapists who listen to and follow the psychological processes, which are sounded in music.

In the previous chapter, it was shown that a lot of music therapists share the idea that the client's thoughts, feelings, and behaviors are echoed in musical processes. As has been worked out, this is so because musical processes and psychological processes are composed of the same amodal temporal and intensity basic forms. The same holds true for processes of change and development. Because musical processes sound the basic processes of the psyche, music therapy is possible. This echoing and sounding has been conceptualized in the concept of "analogy."

As a consequence of the theory of analogy, music therapy methods should be adjusted to the specific characteristics of the disturbance, the handicap, and the individual characteristics of the client. Music therapy for schizophrenic clients should be different from music therapy for depressive or borderline clients and so on, because the protonarrative envelopes of these disturbances are different from each other.

Future research is needed to compare the psychological processes of disturbances and handicaps, and the processes of curing and development, with musical processes. Music therapists with different roots should describe the musical processes used by them in musical and psychological terms. Perhaps then it will be possible to generate a general theory of music therapy that makes possible different methods, with the aim of offering our clients the best music therapy treatment there is.

A PERSPECTIVE FROM ART

In semiotic theory, a distinction is made between the semiotic system, the symbolic system, and the semisymbolic system (Greimas & Courtés, 1979). In the *semiotic* system, there is no link between expression and content. This means that the aesthetic structure does not refer to some other meaning not lying in the aesthetic form itself. In the *symbolic* system, the elements of the aesthetic structure are connected to content outside the aesthetic structure, just like traffic signs and words that point to meanings outside the signs and words themselves. In the *semisymbolic* system, there is not a symbolic connection between the aesthetic structure and content outside, but content is deduced from the formal aspects within the aesthetic structure itself. For music therapy, the semisymbolic system is an interesting perspective, because it gives attention to the arrangements of aesthetic elements in form and the meaning of these arrangements.

In semiology, the process of reasoning to find the correspondence of form and content is called analogizing; the correspondence itself is called a homology, a sameness in structural relatedness of elements. Essential in this way of reasoning is that it is possible to derive content from relationships of form elements; it is not necessary to recognize elements as symbols or signs of phenomena. The aesthetic form—the relationship of aesthetic elements—in itself is content. There is content "inside" the aesthetic. Thus, the way form elements are grouped together gives meaning.

Let me give you an example of how such an analysis of a work of art takes place. In his work on Paul Klee, Thürlemann (1982) analyzes how in Klee's painting *Pflanzen-Analytisches* (1932) the arrangement of abstract elements gives way to meaning. At the top of the canvas, there are three elements arranged vertically and closely connected to each other. At the bottom, three elements are arranged aslant, one of them disconnected from the two other elements. In the middle, all three elements are connected to each other; the constellation is slightly aslant. What the painting tells us, from the semiologist's point of view, is that from the top of the canvas to the bottom there is a "development," a "turn" from vertical to aslant, and a change in elements from being closely connected to each other to being "free." Concepts such as "development," "turn," and "liberation" are meanings connected to the relationships of form elements. If we apply this analytic perspective to music therapy, a client in music therapy can be described as a person who expresses himself in a musical form, which has psychological meaning derived from the way the form elements are arranged.

This perspective differs from the symbolic analysis. When the music therapist understands music as a *symbolic system*, he interprets rhythms, melodies, and sounds like traffic signs. This is close to the Freudian and Jungian way of handling symbols. Freud (1987) found out that in dreams, objects such as a stick, a tree, or a knife can symbolize the male sexual organ. Baskets and cabinets can symbolize the female body. Jung (1985) tells us that the snake can symbolize the unconscious; the fire, the transformation; and the star, the transcendent wholeness. Correspondingly, a rhythm, a melody, or a sound can symbolize a person or a thing. Priestley (1994a) for instance describes how a gong symbolized a child's mother, and a glissando on the xylophone, a horrible lady.

The symbolic system, however, gives us meaning that lies outside the music, not the psychological meaning that is sounded in the present musical form. Music in music therapy is not a city map with traffic signs and symbols. Even when a distinction is made between sign and symbol, see Kristeva (1970), the symbol having a more transcendent meaning, this does not alter the function of the symbol. As the sign, the symbol connects the symbolic representation with a context of meaning outside the representation. For instance, for socialists, the color red is a symbol—it connects a visual representation to ideas of society. These ideas cannot be found inside the color red itself. To know which transcendent ideas this color represents, you have to learn about the connection of the color and the context it points to.

On the contrary, in the *semisymbolic system* this is different. There are no traffic signs or symbols that connect representations with meanings from outside. Meaning in the semisymbolic system comes from within, and is connected to the structure of the representation itself. When traveling in the "musical city of Self," one is not looking at traffic signs or symbols, but at the structure of the city map itself—not as a work of art, but as a musical structure that sounds the structure of the Self.

The expression of the client's Self in music shows us the form of Self, sounded in the form of music. The client's musical form is different from the work of the artist, because the work of the artist is guided by an artistic point of view, which he wants to communicate. He is communicating in art about art, like Jasper Johns asking himself and communicating to his audience, "How do you make a work of art?" On the contrary, the client is not developing art motifs he wants to communicate to others, not using an artistic point of view when expressing his Self. When the client uses an artistic point of view, he withdraws from his Self. Music therapy enables the client to be guided by his inner personal motifs, not by motifs of art. The client then becomes an artist of his Self, sounding the musical form of his Self. The music therapist as the semiologist "understands" the narrative of the client's musical form and "reads" musical form as psychological content, asking himself, "What psychological content can be heard in the client's musical form?"

Before, I raised the idea that all arts therapies might benefit from the theory of analogy, which is grounded in Stern's developmental psychology. I also am convinced that this holds true for the contribution semiology can make to the arts therapies.

THERAPY BEYOND WORDS: PERSONAL CHANGE BY ANALOGOUS EXPERIENCES

A human being is an integrated biological, neurological, psychological, behavioral, and social phenomenon. Therapy means helping a person to transform his old integrated being into a new one. In today's health care world, there are many specialists who focus on parts of the human being. There is the physical doctor, who communicates with the human body by means of chemicals to influence the biological processes and enhance the person's biological balance. The verbal psychotherapist uses words as a communicative medium to help the person to express experiences that can be put into verbal labels.

The psychoanalyst helps to increase consciousness of the "inside"; the behaviorist focuses on changing the "outside" of the psyche. Several decades earlier, humanistic psychotherapy was introduced as a third force, which concentrates on self-actualizing tendencies. All schools of therapy use words as the most prominent medium in therapy.

Although arts therapies also make use of words, I would like to hold to the idea of a "therapy beyond words." Using words in therapy on the one hand can be very close to real life. The content of the words is able to signify directly personal problems and therefore help coping. On the other hand, words can be frightening. A human being can be confronted and become upset when putting his personal problems into words. Words tell him directly who he is. Words can be "definite"; they "fix reality," steal perspective from future, and lead to fixations in the past.

It is the human's fate to live and to reflect on his living, but sometimes it seems as if it would be better not to reflect and tell ourselves who we are. When a person does not reflect on his problems, it may seem as if they are not there. Unfortunately, neither neglecting nor suppressing one's problems leads to health. We need to "express" our inner being. Freud's discovery that the unconscious uses symbols to express indirectly what cannot be put into words directly shows on the one hand how frightening denotative words can be, on the other hand the human drive to express even what is difficult to express.

Whereas the content of words on the one hand can point directly to our problems, on the other hand words are distanced from experience. Words are digital denominators of experiences; they signify an experience, and "talk about" experience. Because words are not actions, they are not experiences themselves—they are labels for experiences. To "know" a mood, we need to experience the mood, we need to be in the "action" of the mood. The word "mood" only points to the mood; it can evoke it, but it is not analogous to it.

When reading a book, the reader, by means of association, evokes internal experiences. However, reading the book is not taking part as an actor in the book. There is no "real" action; there is an action in fantasy. Nobody can learn to play the piano merely by reading a book about how to play the piano. People can become inspired, can enjoy a book, can move through fantasies and dream states and thus have experiences. But a book changes only one domain of our being: our "knowing about" life through fantasy and dream state. Life itself is full of action, and evolving ourselves into action is life. Thus, a book has to be transformed into actions, which are accompanied by vitality affects.

Therapeutic change cannot occur by merely reading and talking about change. The arts therapies offer therapy by means of actions. In the arts therapies, experiences are evoked by means of actions. The therapeutic act is not just cognition or emotion or behavior. All aspects of the person in an integrated way are put into the therapeutic act; there is cognition, emotion, movement, social interaction, and so on. In the therapeutic act, the person is experiencing a life situation in which he is involved completely as a person.

The therapeutic act can be preceded and followed by words—words even can be used during the therapeutic act itself—but the essence of arts therapies is that there is experience in acting out. This experience is an analogous experience; it is not life reality as is outside therapy, or a mere reflection of this outside life reality. The arts therapies offer a context where actions are different from outside life reality but experiences that are evoked by these actions are real.

In the arts therapies, clients are acting in a musical, dramatic, art, and movement space. In these actions, cognition, emotion, movement, social interaction, and other domains of the integrated human being are expressed. In the music, the dramatic scene, the painting, or the movement, the client is expressing himself as he expresses himself in other life situations. The characteristics of the arts materials help him to express himself; they also offer opportunities of change. When, for example, there is a change in the musical act, then there is a change in the intra- and/or interpersonal process.

This brings us to an essential aspect of human life. How do we express our person? By telling how we feel or by showing our feelings through the song of our voice, the movement of our body, the color of our dress, the way we play our roles as a partner, a teacher, a child? An anecdote about a spiritual guru tells us that he did not tell about the essence of life, but showed his students how to tie their shoes.

Today, there is much talk "about" many things. The world of words and talk seems to be the "real" world, just as the logos of multinational companies seem to represent human experiences and values. Computers are used as metaphors for human beings, and words are used as labels for "understanding" human experience. I think that the actions in the arts therapies can give us more of a felt sense about each other and ourselves than words, figures, and logos combined.

Chapter Seven

DEFINING AND REDEFINING THE CORE CATEGORY OF ANALOGY[1]

INTRODUCTION

Now we have come to the last step of the research journey that started in Chapter Five. In this chapter, I will give a definition of analogy in which all the previous conclusions will be integrated. The properties of the core category will be described in detail. Also, a glossary gives an overview of related but different concepts that have been discussed in the previous chapters and some new concepts. In the end, the idea of a transformational language will be discussed and an example of this language will be presented.

DEFINING ANALOGY

In this part, I will define the properties of the core category of analogy. To begin with, it should be clear that the core category of analogy contains two subcategories. The first is the analogy in diagnosis; the second is the analogy in treatment. The former subcategory refers to the similarity between forms of music expressed by the client and forms of feeling that characterize his disturbance or handicap. The latter subcategory refers to forms of music that sound changes of forms of feeling that improve health.

There also can be made a distinction between *specific* and *nonspecific* analogies. Nonspecific means that a client acts in music therapy as he acts elsewhere, but this action is not in music (for instance, when a client does not participate in activities or stops activities very quickly. This can happen with all sorts of activities). Specific means that the analogy occurs in the music (a client acts in music as he acts elsewhere). The following definition of analogy refers to specific analogies in diagnosis and treatment

Analogy can be defined with a set of theses:

---

[1]Parts of this chapter have been presented during conferences and were prepared in earlier publications.

- Music therapy differs from the real-life context outside music therapy because in the real-life context a person normally does not express himself or communicates by means of musical actions. Therefore, an analogy is not a replica because psychological processes are not replicated exactly, but expressed in another medium (the music).
- The difference from the real-life context, which is available because analogy is not a replica, makes it possible that music therapy can be experienced as a safe, experimental space, or a field of play in which daily rules are bracketed.
- Although this experimental space is not identical to the real-life context, in music therapy the psychological phenomena (thoughts, feelings, and behaviors) that are experienced are not different from real-life context.
- The musical process in music therapy is an analogy of the psychological process because there is no dualism between the musical form and the form of feeling as there is between a symbolic form and the psychological process it refers to. When there is analogy, musical forms are no symbols of what is not manifest. Because the musical form does not refer to something else, there is no need for interpretation.
- The analogous musical process has embodied meaning and means what is manifest. The analogous musical processes are what it is about. Being-in-the-music is being-in-the-experience.
- Analogy is semisymbolic; it gives attention to the arrangements of musical form elements and the meaning of these arrangements. Psychological meaning (content) can be derived from the relationships of form elements.
- In analogy, there is a (semisymbolic) sameness of the basic parameters of musical and psychological phenomena. Because of this basic sameness, music affects us directly without the need for an intermediary process of remembering, thinking, associating, and imagining. Analogy offers a primary type of knowledge, intimate knowledge that is intuitive, nonintermediary, nonsubstitutional, nondualistic, direct, and nonabstract. Music is "a language of immediacy."
- Analogies occur because of the similarity of the temporal and intensity patterns that is shared by the forms of feeling and the forms of music. It is possible to describe musical forms with the same dynamic kinetic terms that describe vitality affects.

In music there is a dramatic line of tension (that) is invariably synchronous with the temporal feeling shape (protonarrative envelope).

- In music therapy, the client by means of his musical expression makes manifest his *music of the Self.* He expresses himself in the music in the same way he expresses himself in other contexts and by other media of expression. Unhealthy thoughts, feelings, and behaviors come to sound in the musical play and musical choice of a client.
- In music therapy, pathological protonarrative envelopes become expressed in sound and are changed into healthy envelopes.
- Because a person is able to perceive (amodal) temporal and intensity patterns in different processes and modalities of expression, it is possible to express and perceive intra- and interpersonal forms of feeling in patterns of music.
- The client can express his own feelings and the feelings of others by the transfer of forms of feeling into musical forms of perception, and by the retransfer of the musical forms of perception back into forms of feeling.
- Analogy is not limited to specific processes but can be applied to many psychological intra- and interpersonal and musical processes.
- Music therapy is the appropriate form of therapy when musical processes can be initiated that are composed of patterns that are equal to those psychological patterns that lead to health with a particular population of clients.
- To make sure that there is analogy each time, the analogy should be corroborated by the client's and the music therapist's experience.
- Analogy is a core category because many music therapists, who have their roots in many different therapeutic schools and work with many different populations of clients, use it.
- Analogy acts as a core category, includes other therapeutic categories, and has a central position between other categories

From this definition of analogy, and the previous chapters, it should be clear that analogy is a psychological concept that is grounded on the empirical evidence that the temporal and intensity patterns within the forms of perception and the forms of feeling are equal and experienced as such.

As has been put forward in previous chapters, analogy stresses the sameness between processes (of perception and feeling) that can be compared to each other. Therefore, it excludes all sorts of mystical, magical, esoteric, metaphysical, quasi-philosophical, and other speculative concepts, which connect phenomena that, in their essential characteristics, cannot be compared to each other.

Speculative concepts suggest that music can be therapeutic, because of superficial correspondences between nonpsychological phenomena—for example, correspondences between mathematical relationships of cosmic, physical objects, musical intervals, harmonies, and the human body (for a critique see Summer, 1996, and Hartogh, 2002). Speculative concepts are nonpsychological and based on ideas taken from the Pythagorean School of philosophy; Boethius's idea of correspondence between musica mundana, musica instrumentalis, and musica instrumentalis; and Rudolf Steiner's anthroposophical linear equations between human processes (thinking, feeling, willing), and music (melody, harmony, rhythm, meter).

These sorts of ideas lack psychological reason and empirical evidence, and connect phenomena to each other by means of irrelevant features. Many objections are obvious. I will give some examples: The mere correspondence between mathematical forms (for instance between planets, intervals, and the human body) cannot explain why one object influences another. The statement that there is "harmony" in music (consonant chords) and "harmony" in the human being (psychological well-being) cannot explain why music influences the human being.

At their best, these speculative ideas are metaphors that give us a poetic idea of the numinous power of music. But the problems with these concepts are that they are presented and sold as therapeutic evidence.

Authors such as Hartogh (2002) criticize these metaphorical rationales, and I strongly agree with their critiques. However, Hartogh holds a very outdated idea of analogy and equates analogy with metaphor. As a result of this, he suggests that there should be differentiation between metaphor/analogy on the one hand and homology on the other hand. However, in a more updated meaning of analogy, analogy is different from metaphor and is equal to homology. As we saw before, this holds true for Stern's developmental psychology, and in semiology, where the process of analogizing leads to homology.

In the next section, the difference between analogy and metaphor will be addressed further.

A GLOSSARY OF CONCEPTS

After the journey into literature, developmental psychology, and semiology in the previous chapters, and before going into music therapy clinical practice more deeply, let me summarize by defining several concepts and at the same time distinguish these concepts from the concept of analogy. In previous passages, I put forward that it is important to differentiate between analogy, metaphor, and symbol. Because these concepts refer to very different psychological processes, they give way to different methods of music therapy and rationales. And there are more concepts that we should consider.

When there is a *replica*, something looks exactly the same as the object it represents. Take, for example, the little statue on your desk, which is a real statue rebuilt in small form. A replica also can be built in exactly the same physical size as the original. For instance, it is possible to rebuild a 17th-century ship as big as the original. Then the rebuilt ship is not the original, but an exact copy. In music, a replica would mean that a musical event is rebuilt exactly, when for example a lady in the same outfit and with the same voice sings songs in the manner of Marlene Dietrich.

A *representation* refers to the portrayal, picture, or image of an object. In visual art in previous centuries, the artists created on their canvas representations, images of the real things. Photographers take pictures of all kinds of things; the cinema, television, and the computer give us virtual realities on screens. These representations are not replicas because there is no physical relationship between the representation and the object, but only a representation on canvas, paper, or screen. In musical art, in the past "Tonmalerei" ("drawing with sounds") has been introduced. When using Tonmalerei, the sounds of an object or event are not replicated by using exactly the same sounds, but by means of instrumental sounds that somehow can suggest the sounds of the original object. A well-known example is the thunder in Beethoven's Pastorale symphony, which is suggested by the use of orchestral sounds. In music therapy, in a thematic improvisation sounds can be used to represent the sounds of real events (an airplane, the rain, and so on).

A *semirepresentation* in some aspects sounds like the object that is represented, but it is no complete representation—the representation is something else, too. For instance, the male sexual organ in a dream, being represented by a stick, is a semirepresentation. Because of the dynamics of dreamwork—as we know, from Freud—suppressed content is not represented in full. In a dream, the sexual wish will be disguised and the object (for example, the phallus) will be represented by something that might look like a phallus but also can represent something else, such as a stick. Although the stick in a dream in some aspects looks like the phallus, it also represents something else: a real stick.

In music therapy, for instance, strong dynamics can represent the vocal outbursts of the father, and traumatic experiences that were evoked by these outbursts, but strong dynamics can also represent traffic sounds. These dynamics somehow express the original experience, and at the same time disguise it.

As has been discussed in several previous sections, in the *symbol* there is no direct correspondence between its form and the object it refers to. As Aigen (1995a) puts it: In symbolization, there is a "dualism" between the symbol and the object. A symbol refers to something without resembling it; the symbol does not mirror the object. For example, the snake symbolizing the unconscious does not resemble the unconscious, because the unconscious in no way looks like a snake. As has been put forward in previous chapters, the color red is a symbol for socialism, but the color itself has no characteristics of socialism. Because there is no resemblance in these cases, besides the symbol and the object we need a third (indirect) cognitive aspect, a link between the symbol and the object. Thus there is a need for "interpretation."[2]

What has been said about the symbol holds true also when a *metaphor* is used. The metaphor, as well as the symbol, is different from analogy.[3] By means of a metaphor, characteristics of one object are described with characteristics of another object. As Dissanayake (1996, p. 169) notes: "...metaphors allow us to understand and experience one thing in terms of another ..." By means of a metaphor, the camel can be described as "the ship of the desert"; the unconscious, as "the caves of our psyche"; and people, as "... deep and shallow, narrow and wide, hard and soft, as well as bright (light) and dull (dark) ..." (Dissanayake, 1996, p. 174).

The camel is described with characteristics of the ship; the psyche, with characteristics of a mountain with caves; and people, with all sorts of physical terms. However, the structure of the camel in no way is like the structure of a ship. Like a ship, the camel takes its passengers on a long trip through an uninhabited part of the world. When using a metaphor, we make use of a cognitive operation that connects characteristics of the ship to the camel. The cognitive operation tells us that the camel and the ship both traverse long distances. This resemblance makes it possible to make associations between the camel and characteristics of the ship, which of course gives us a broader view on this animal. In this case, it is the shared functional characteristics, not the equality of structure, that we are talking about.

---

[2]See Chapter Eight for a discussion on the link of semiotic and symbolic aspects in Kristeva's sense, connected to the case of Edward.

[3]Stern sees the nonverbal metaphor and analogy both as differentiated from the verbal symbol. In his opinion, there is a development from imitation through analogy and metaphor to symbol.

In the same way, we use a cognitive operation of association when we talk about the "caves of the psyche." A mountain has caves that go deep into it, we do not know what is in it, and this not knowing makes us anxious. Our psyche does not have caves, but we can say that just as a mountain has caves, our psyche has thoughts and feelings that are hidden, which we do not know and are afraid of. The caves, as well as the hidden thoughts and feelings, evoke anxiety because of something we do not know. The metaphor makes it possible to understand our psyche with the help of the characteristics of the caves. But, of course, the structure of our psyche is not like the structure of caves.

The difference between analogy and metaphor needs little more attention. If we want to explain why a metaphor is experienced, we need the analogy. I described how in the metaphor of "harmony" the client makes a cognitive connection between his psyche and the music. However, it is also possible that the client, without the cognitive belief system, experiences directly the harmony of music as psychological well-being. Musical harmony exists when there is no tension between tones, which is perceived as the music being in rest, without a drive to move to a solution. There is the perception of a temporal form being at rest. When the psyche is "in harmony," there is no conflict between the person's needs, which should be released. This lack of conflict, and the lack of a drive for solution of the conflict, is experienced as a form of feeling. Because the temporal form of music, which is perceived, and the form of feeling are equal, musical harmony directly can be experienced as psychological "harmony." The musical form has a protonarrative envelope, which is equal to the form of feeling.

The history of music therapy theory is full of sentences such as "A disturbance means that the psyche is in disharmony; musical harmony can restore the disharmony of the psyche" and so on. This sentence includes two connections that should be researched. First, there is a connection made between the disturbance and the concept of "disharmony." When doing so, one should ask whether this diagnosis is valid, and if it is, whether it gives enough information about the client's problem. The second connection is made between the "harmony of the psyche" and musical harmony. With both connections, we should be aware of the difference between the metaphor and equality in structure.

When a metaphor is used, the metaphor itself gives no psychological evidence. It is the client's experience of the metaphor that counts. In music therapy, we use an image (disharmony in music) that by means of a cognitive operation helps us to understand something else (the psychological disturbance). We should not use the metaphor literally, as a valid structural description of the disturbance or as an adequate rationale for the effect of music therapy. We should not confuse this cognitive operation with a psychological explanation—as in analogy—that describes the structural relationships of music and psyche.

The metaphor, as it is used in therapy, is an image, which can be therapeutic because it enables a cognitive operation that leads to more understanding of a psychological phenomenon. The metaphor is therapeutic when the client is suggestible for the metaphor and believes that he is in "disharmony" and that he can be cured by musical "harmony." It is the client's metaphorical imagination, his belief system, which makes it possible to experience a musical resolution "as if" it were a psychological one. And because of the belief system, the client indeed can experience psychological resolution when listening to musical resolution.

The point with symbols and metaphors is that while they can be very helpful in music therapy, music therapists should be conscious about the psychological processes they are working with. And what is more, when we explain music therapy, symbol, metaphor, and analogy represent different rationales and should not become confused.

When there is *semisymbolism,* there is a correspondence between meaningful, formal aspects of the musical structure and the personal structure. Meaning is derived from the arrangement of musical form elements, not from interpreting musical elements as symbols or signs of phenomena outside the musical structure. In music therapy, the client's music and psyche share formal relationships. The way sounds are grouped together gives formal meaning, which includes psychological meaning as well, because it shows how the person's Self organizes formal elements.

In conclusion, I state that *analogy* is not a replica, not a representation or semirepresentation, not a symbol or metaphor. A musical analogy is not a replication of a musical event; it is not a complete (or partly) re-sounding of sounds by means of music, as in Tonmalerei. There is no dualism between the musical form and its meaning as there is with the symbol, nor a cognitive operation of association as in metaphor. When there is analogy, the person expresses his Self in musical form, in the same way he expresses himself in other modalities, in other contexts, and by other objects.

Let me discuss some theories and concepts of my colleagues and the relationships of these to the concept of analogy.

Analogy is defined by Hesse (1967, quoted by Aigen, 1995c) as having not a physical but a formal relationship. To illustrate this, Aigen gives the example of "resonating ideas." In my opinion, "resonating ideas" is a metaphor like "ship of the desert" and "caves of the psyche." As I said before, a cognitive operation of association is needed that illustrates one phenomenon with characteristics of the other. "Resonating" is a concept from physics referring to an object making sound because it is hit by certain sounds of another object, and both objects share equal sound frequencies. In the case of ideas, there can be agreement. Ideas cannot "resonate" physically as sound frequencies do. By means of association, the resonance of frequencies and the agreement of ideas are linked to each other.

One might question whether the way the word "formal" has been used by Hesse is adequate. When there is analogy, when "musical forms are equal to the forms of feeling," then form is not just a metaphor. Forms of feeling and musical form share the same amodal parameters.

Bonde (in Wigram, Nygaard Pedersen, & Bonde, 2002) develops a theory of music as metaphor, which is based on the psychological equivalence of musical elements as well as the client's presentation of his music experience verbally using metaphor. Bonde gives examples of metaphors that are equal to the examples I gave above (for instance, "the eyes are the mirror of the soul"), and thus uses the same concept of metaphor. He also puts forward that metaphor is a basic tool of cognition, making, for example, associations such as joy equals "up" and sadness equals "down."

He then gives examples of three "psychological levels of music," where in the first example (Pachelbel, "Canon in D"), the basso ostinato is a metaphor for the "good enough father or mother"; in the second example (J.S. Bach, "Passacaglia and Fugue in C Minor," BWV 582), the basso ostinato is a metaphor for "a voice in command"; and in the third example (J.S. Bach, "Crucifixus from Mass in B Minor," BWV 232), the basso ostinato is a metaphor for "the voice of absurdity." All of these examples indeed are metaphors, which for clients come to the fore by a cognitive operation. These types of metaphors can be idiosyncratic or shared. The metaphors are much stronger when they are evoked by clients themselves, as when music therapists introduce them. Of course, it is necessary, as Bonde in his exposé on metaphor concludes, that the GIM therapist be systematically trained in metaphoric music listening, but eventually the clinical validity of the metaphor depends on the client's experience.

Although there will be some overlap of metaphor and analogy, an analogy is more direct, is felt as a form of feeling, and does not use an image as the metaphor does. The link between image and feeling can be vice versa: The music by means of the cognitive operation can evoke the image and then stimulate a form of feeling, or it can be the other way around when the music (by means of analogy) evokes a form of feeling first, which then is associated with the image of the metaphor.

Gregg (1991) introduces a "structural" theory of personality in which he sees an *analogy* between the personality and certain basic structures of music. He states that the Self is a semiotic system that "... by encoding sublime abstractions in concrete symbols, infuses the endlessly fluctuating concrete minutiae of daily life with ontological significance" (Gregg, 1991, p. 46). There is a process of encoding and self-representation, a process of perception and cognition. What Gregg thinks is analogous between the personality and the music is the structural ambiguity, which in musical terms makes two tones of an octave "same" and "different" (perception), which means that in Boring's young-woman/old-woman allusion one can see an old or a young woman (perception), which in ontological terms shows that there is "me" and "not me," and "self" and "other," and, in ethical terms, "good" and "bad" at the same time. He sees an analogy between the inner dialogue of different and opposed parts of the Self and the fugue, in which several voices play inversions and reversals of a single theme. The structural ambiguity is fundamentally cognitive, and Gregg describes the "... primary units of cognition in general ... (and) the primary operations of thought" (Gregg, 1991, p. 47). One could say that he describes the amodal cognitive operations of the Self.

Mulder (1996) also focuses on the example of the fugue and puts forward the *analogy* and *isomorphism* between the structure of the fugue and the novel. In a novel, she says, there can be an entanglement of several persons, as in the fugue there is an entanglement of voices. She shows that Duras's novel has inversions and fusions of characters, as in the fugue there are inversions and fusion of voices. She links the fugato processes to the processes that occur in the so-called Traumarbeit as described by Freud. Mulder constructs a three-part analogy between the structure of the novel (fusion of characters), the structure of the fugue (fusion of voices), and the structure of dreamwork (fusion of unconscious content by means of the fusion of images).

The theories from Bonde, Gregg, and Mulder are theories that have been developed from the perspective of characteristics of music such as the ostinato, the octave relation, and the fugue. The functions of the ostinato, the octave, and the fusion of voices in the fugue are connected to psychological meanings. Bonde explicitly uses the experience of the metaphor as a bridge from music to psyche.

Gregg and Mulder both use the concept of analogy, but the question arises as to whether their concept of analogy is equal to the way it has been described in this book. Gregg describes basic cognitive operations of the Self, and Mulder describes the "techniques" of dreamwork as deduced by Freud. As Hermans (1993) puts forward in his review, Gregg clearly uses music as a metaphor in the study of personality. Gregg's metaphor is a cognitive tool for representing the Self. There is nothing in the Self that sounds like an octave, as is the case in analogy.

Although Mulder refers to an analogy of the primary process of music and psyche, this is different from analogy as defined in this book. A person can experience the fusion of voices in the fugue *as if* it were a fusion of unconscious contents, but this experience needs a process of insight-oriented cognitive decoding and is not the spontaneous "intimate knowledge" that is typical for analogy. When there is analogy, you experience directly the vitality affects and protonarrative envelopes of the psyche in the music. The fusion of voices in the fugue might be able to evoke the experience of the fusion of unconscious contents, but this is not the intuitive, nonintermediary, nonsubstitutional, nondualistic, and direct experience as in analogy. The fusion of voices in the fugue is not an event that directly is perceived and apprehended right away in terms of a dramatic line of tension that is invariably synchronous with a temporal feeling shape (see Stern's protonarrative envelopes). This is because these temporal feeling shapes are built by dynamic, kinetic qualities, such as "surging," "fading away," "fleeting," "explosive," "crescendo," "decrescendo," "bursting," and "drawn out" (Stern), which are characteristic of vitality affects but differ from thematic melodic structures that are present in the fugue.

There are several other authors who refer to *form*. Aldridge (1989) introduces (besides analogy) the concept of *isomorphism*, referring to a strong connection between musical form, biological form (heart rate, blood pressure, breathing pattern), and personality characteristics (Type A behavior). He describes music as a play of patterned frequencies within a matrix of time, and people as "... beings in the world who are patterned frequencies in time" (Aldridge, 1989, p. 95). Aldridge mainly refers to bodily rhythms such as being awake and sleeping, breath, heartbeat, and so on, which have their own pitch, timbre, and duration.

Representatives from the German school for *morphological* music therapy, such as, for instance, Tüpker (1988/1996), focus on analogies between psychological and musical forms. They describe music and psyche by means of six factors, based on the psychology of Salber (1965). Salber describes psychological processes as the forming and transforming of Gestalts. The six factors that constitute these processes are: appropriation ("Aneignung"), metamorphosis ("Umbildung"), influence ("Einwirkung"), arrangement ("Anordnung"), unfolding ("Ausbreitung"), and equipment ("Ausrüstung").

"Appropriation" means adopting something or becoming adopted by something; "metamorphosis" means changing or being changed; "influence" is to cause something or be caused by something; "arrangement" means being limited by structure or finding a structure; "unfolding" refers to transcending experiences; and, finally, "equipment" refers to the resources that make it possible to do something.

In morphological psychology, music therapists found a fruitful theoretical concept to prove that what happens in the music is the same as what happens in the psyche. Therefore, these music therapists claim that the musical improvisation is the prototype of the forming and transforming of the psyche. The strong point is that there is an analogy between the music and the psyche. Morphologists argue that these six factors form the basics of psychological functioning. From this, it is deduced that focusing in treatment on these factors will influence the psyche and influence the disturbance. But somehow this rationale is reductionistic, reducing psychological processes and disturbances to six factors and concluding that when these factors will be influenced, the psyche will be cured.

Sure, disturbances can be described by the six factors of morphology, and they can be used in therapy. However, one should raise the question whether the Gestalt factors describe the psyche in full. Indeed, it is possible to describe the psyche by means of these Gestalt factors, but can these Gestalt factors describe the core characteristics of all psychological processes and disturbances? These factors can only describe some aspects of the psychological processes and disturbances, which are much more differentiated and complex. Thus, I am not convinced that all disturbances can be described and treated merely by using these six factors. When influencing the Gestalt factors the person will change, but will the disturbance be cured? When looking at the six factors, one also might ask whether they describe musical improvisations in full. Is it possible to describe the essence of all sorts of musical improvisation by means of these Gestalt factors?

Pavlicevic (1997), when referring to semiology and the work of Pierce (1932) and Nattiez (1990), makes a distinction between music as symbol, music as icon, and music as index. Her way of reasoning is very close to mine when she is telling us that the manner in which the symbol relates to the object is the central issue.

As has been discussed before, a symbol does not resemble its object. This is different with the *icon*. An icon somehow resembles the object to which it refers. As Pavlicevic points out, the word "cat" is symbolic, whereas a (representational) drawing of a cat is iconic. The icon is equal to the representation I discussed before and to Tonmalerei in music ("drawing by means of sound").

One interesting question is whether the concept of the icon can, as Pavlicevic seems to suggest, be used when we talk about tension and relaxation in music. Can we say that tension and relaxation in music are an icon of tension and relaxation in human feeling? An icon is something that visually or auditorily resembles an object. The icon gives us a more or less concrete visual or auditory representation of an object. We might say that an icon gives us the "figure" of the object. In the case of emotions, this would be a drawing of somebody who is angry, or the sounds made by somebody who is angry. Thus, an icon gives us the "figure" of the categorical affects (see Stern, 1985). However the process of tension and relaxation in anger describes the vitality affect of this categorical feeling, we might say that it is the amodal "background" of the emotion. Therefore, I would like to distinguish between the icon as the superficial representation or semirepresentation of an object, and the analogy as the semisymbolic formal structure of the object.

Pavlicevic describes two ways in which tension and relaxation in music are connected to tension and relaxation of human feeling, the "indirect" and the "direct" way. She addresses the same aspect that I put forward when discussing the "third" cognitive aspect, which refers to an indirect cognitive operation of association, which in symbol and metaphor makes a link between two phenomena. Following Stern, she refers to Langer's (1951) idea that music reflects the *morphology of feelings* (patterns of tension and resolution, dynamic shifts).

Langer's theory seems to be very close to vitality affects as described by Stern, and to analogy, when she states that music does not reflect specific emotions but their morphological patterns, the properties of feelings. But Langer's view is "indirect" when she supposes an act of recognition, or as Stern puts it, some sort of contemplative mode, which recognizes art as form of feeling and transcends the direct involvement with feeling. When, according to Langer, people *recognize* their forms of feeling in the forms of music, this happens by means of a cognitive operation.

On the contrary, when there is a "direct" connection between music and psyche—Pavlicevic calls this connection "music as index"—music is not recognized as an aspect of us, but music and feeling are an "organic pair." If Pavlicevic's "organic pair" is not interpreted as a purely biological/neurological inscription in the mind, but as a direct, nondiscursive, intuitive, tacit "understanding" of similarity, then the concept of music as index is very close to the concept of analogy, which has been defined as the (semisymbolic) sameness of the amodal characteristics of the forms of feeling and the forms of music.

As Pavlicevic puts it: "… my mind already 'knows' what 'sagging/dragging' is/looks like/sounds like, and my mind is receptive to being stimulated by the 'sagging and dragging' in the music" (Pavlicevic, 1997, p. 31). I agree that music affects us directly, "… bypassing symbolic meaning, and, to some extent, iconic signification …" (p. 32). If we do not know its symbolic meaning, if we do not recognize what it sounds like, music nevertheless affects us.

No theory of symbolic association, conditioning or representation ever can fully explain the effect of music (therapy). The influence of music on man can be explained fully neither by an arbitrary individual or collective link made between the object of music and some meaning, nor because in the past a stimulus-response link has been established, nor because music sounds like the manifest sounds in man's environment. To become affected by music, there is no need for a "signifying agent." However, as music therapists, we should be cautious with the conclusion that music as such is therapeutic. By means of theory and research, we need to describe which musical processes are analogous to psychological processes. If we do not, then we will not be able to prove why music therapy is more than "just making music," and not be able to explain its therapeutic significance. Saying that there is a direct link between music and psyche is only the beginning of a theory of music therapy. We need to describe musical processes as vitality affects and research which musical processes should be used with clients in treatment.

We should not presume that the innate "organic pair" of music and feeling is sufficient to help the client as a medicine would. The client should experience the forms of music as his forms of feeling. The client should not just intuitively, but also, as therapy proceeds, more consciously experience his Self in the music. (This experience is different from the cognitive operation we discussed before; it is not a recognition by argument, but a recognition by immediate experience.)

Remember one of Priestley's clients, who, when listening to his musical improvisation, has an "AHA-Erlebnis" and reacts by saying:

> "This is me. I am really like that inside. I pretend to be so strong with my great voice singing and shouting and smashing windows but really I am very weak." (Priestley, 1994b, p. 238).

Or take some sentences from my own cases in which the clients reached insights, such as "Playing the piano is like my life" (Smeijsters, 1999a; Smeijsters & Van den Hurk, 1999) and "Interaction in music is similar to interaction at home" (Smeijsters & Storm, 1997/1998).

OBJECTIONS

Let us pick up some possible objections to the theory of analogy. One objection is that a person does not express in music who he is, but who he can be. In this view, music is seen as a domain that offers new possibilities because musical experience is different from experience in daily life. Music therapists sometimes tell us that the client reacts completely differently from what had been expected. The argument that the client behaves differently in music therapy is not really in conflict with the theory of analogy. When the client behaves differently, this shows how different he can be. In both cases, music sounds his psyche.

A second objection would be that playing a piece of Mozart is only a weak expression of the person who plays it. And indeed, when there is a lot of precomposed structure, there is little opportunity for individual personal expression, although there is in the way of performing. There is more personal expression when, as in music therapy, there is free improvisation. Therefore, musical improvisation has been called the midwife of personal expression and growth in music therapy.

On the other hand, musical structures—self-made songs, popular and classical precomposed musical pieces—offer musical forms that sound forms of feelings as well. In receptive music therapy such Guided Imagery and Music, the imagery is evoked because the precomposed music evokes forms of feeling and through these stimulates the process of association. Thus, the cognitive operation is enabled because of the musical form.

A third objection can be that when intrapersonal processes are not only expressed in musical actions but in other actions as well, why should there be music therapy? In the first part of this chapter, I made the distinction between *specific* and *nonspecific* analogies.

As we explored in previous chapters, the link between vitality affects and musical forms is very tight. Both forms are described by means of the same words, which show that the musical and psychological dynamic processes are formed by the same amodal parameters. Thus, music and music therapy, because of these parameters, have therapeutic significance.

A fourth objection is that there is not yet enough scientific evidence that there is transfer from changes in music therapy to changes in other life domains. This objection of course holds true for every sort of therapy. In the case of analogy, we expect that a change in the amodal characteristics of intra- and interpersonal experiences and behaviors will result in changes in different contexts. For example, when the client learns to be less impulsive in the musical interaction, we expect that he will be less impulsive in verbal communication. Because the protonarrative envelopes of the musical and verbal interactions are the same, there can synchronously be a change in verbal interaction when there is in musical interaction. However, learning often is limited by its context, so mostly what has been learned in music therapy should be transferred more explicitly to other contexts. The music therapist, or the psychotherapist, should focus on these nonmusical contexts, and help the client to cope with it. Because the client has learned in music therapy already to reduce his impulses, learning in another (real-life) context will be much easier.

TOWARD AN INTERMEDIARY LANGUAGE

Ansdell (1995, p. 179) uses the concept of "intrinsic interpretation" when describing how, in an improvisation, the music therapist makes a musical response. The music therapist reacts on the musical process. He does not translate music into "another thing" (for instance, an image) on which he reacts, Ansdell tells us.

Although I agree with this line of thought, I would like to stress that the "direct" expression of the client in music and the "intrinsic interpretation" of the client's musical expression by the music therapist should not be misunderstood as a purely musical process. The musical process and the musical analysis of this process need to be linked to psychological "meaning." I put forward that this meaning is not symbolic or metaphoric. On the other hand, this meaning is more than purely musical and should give us more understanding about the process than musical analysis is able to give us. I agree with Ansdell that psychological meaning should not be the result of interpretation, which seeks latent meanings behind manifest musical expressions. But we need a link between the musical process and psychological process, which, as in analogy, connects the musical forms directly to forms of feeling. Therefore, we need a new type of musical analysis in which the musical and the psychological are integrated, or as Pavlicevic puts it, are an "organic pair."

To give words to the new type of musical analysis we need an intermediary language, between the language of psychology/psychotherapy, which uses psychological concepts, and the musical language, which uses musical concepts. Bengtsson (1973) points out that the nonverbal cannot be "translated" into the verbal. The same problem occurs when music therapists try to translate musical language into psychological language. Somehow there seems to be a gap between the musical score and the psychological meaning. In my opinion, this gap will continue to exist when one tries to translate two distinct languages into each other.

One of the handicaps of music therapy seems to be that, on the one hand, there is the traditional musical analysis and language, which describes the musical process, and on the other hand there is the language from psychology, psychopathology, and psychotherapy, which describes the human psyche. As long as music therapy has existed, there has been the problem of translating one language into the other. One group of music therapists, who stress that music is an art, use the musical language and have difficulties in explaining why the musical is psychological. A second group of music therapists, with their roots in psychotherapy, use the psychological language and have difficulties in showing how the psychological is sounded in the music.

The intermediary language we need should use words that at the same time have musical and psychological meaning. The words include the forms of music and the forms of feeling, and make a bridge between the purely musical and the purely psychological languages. For example, a word such as "variation" can be an intermediary between the musical language and psychological language. This same word tells us something about the musical process and the personal process; it is a musical/psychological concept, which assesses the music and the person as well.

Bruscia (1987) developed Improvisation Assessment Profiles such as the "variation profile," "integration profile," "tension profile," "congruence profile," "salience profile," and "autonomy profile," which can be part of the intermediary language. Bruscia uses the profiles to draw "... analogies with a wide variety of psychological theories ..." (Bruscia, 1987, p. 411). As with the theory of analogy I propose in this book, Bruscia's profiles are free from a specific theoretical orientation.

He describes three levels of interpretation: 1) the analogy between musical behavior and the performance of tasks outside of music; 2) the analogy between musical functioning and other nonmusical areas of functioning; and 3) music as projection of the personality, as sign of the conscious or unconscious. The third level of interpretation is existential or psychoanalytic, while the first and the second are close to analogy as described in this book.

At that time, the link with Stern's psychology and the bridge between the forms of music and the forms of feeling by means of the amodal parameters of both had not been made yet. Nevertheless, these profiles surely can be part of the intermediary language in a way that the musical and psychological are integrated as I discussed before.

Bruscia also described 64 clinical techniques that the music therapist can use. These techniques include concepts that can be part of the intermediary language. See, for example, concepts such as "imitating," "making spaces," "interjecting," "introducing change," "differentiating," "intensifying," "calming," "pausing," "receding," and many more (Bruscia, 1987, pp. 535–537). These concepts are not typically musical, and can refer to musical behavior as well as nonmusical behavior (for instance, they can describe verbal and nonverbal communication). Bruscia's techniques are about the music therapist's behavior, but with some alterations they can describe the client's behavior.

In Bruscia's 64 clinical techniques, besides the intermediary (analog) concepts, there are two types of concepts that are different. Some concepts clearly belong to the musical language, such as "rhythmic grounding," "tonal centering," "sharing instruments," "modulating," "conducting," "rehearsing," "performing," and so on. Other concepts belong to psychological theories, concepts such as "holding," "integrating," "free associating," "projecting," "splitting," and so on. In my opinion, it would be wise to differentiate between these three types of concepts (the intermediary, the musical, and the psychological).

Words used by Stern, such as "... surging, fading away, fleeting, explosive, crescendo, decrescendo, bursting, drawn out, and so on" (Stern, 1985, p. 54), all can be used in the intermediary language. Music and the psyche both can be "explosive." The word "explosive" at the same time is a musical and psychological concept, which on the one hand can make a bridge to musical parameters such as tempo, rhythm, and dynamics, and on the other hand can make a bridge to psychological concepts such as, for example, an outburst of anger.

The strong point in morphological music therapy is that the musical process clearly is described as an analogy of the psychological process. The language of morphological music therapy is an intermediary language that can be applied equally to music and the psyche. The concepts that are used when describing improvisation do not need to be translated into psychological language. Morphologists themselves argue that when using this method, problems of translation do not exist at all. However, as has been discussed before, although the six factors of morphology can be part of the intermediary language, we need more words to describe disturbances and therapeutic processes to reduce problems of translation.

The concept of *dynamic form* used by Pavlicevic (1990) at first glance might be confusing because she uses words such as "dynamics" and "form," which in music have specific meaning. But, these words should not be understood merely as musical terms. Pavlicevic refers to Stern (1985), who, as I described before, uses terms such as "dynamic" to describe the qualities of the vitality affects. Then dynamic form, as used by Pavlicevic, signifies amodal patterns. The dynamic form is amodal and goes beyond the merely musical and psychological modality; it is neither purely musical nor purely psychological. She defines dynamic form as being distinct from both musical form and form of feeling, but containing both:

> "It is a form whose features are not exclusively musical, but neither are they exclusively emotional. [It is a] … musical/emotional form, which is a statement of the Self in the world …" (Pavlicevic, 1995, p. 55-56).

Because, as described by Pavlicevic, the dynamic forms include both music and emotional life, there is an analogy between musical and emotional life. Although in the strict sense there is no "interpretation," there is psychological meaning.

To conclude, concepts such as analogy, dynamic form, and those from morphology give music therapy an independent position and at the same time bridge the gap between the musical and psychological language.

A SEMIOTIC PERSPECTIVE FROM MUSIC THERAPY CLINICAL PRACTICE

In a previous section, I discussed the contribution of semiology to music therapy. Now, let me give a semiotic perspective with a case from clinical practice in which I tried to develop an intermediary language.

The improvisation of the client will be described as a musical form, in which the client has arranged musical elements. From this musical form, meaning will be derived and be expressed in intermediary words, which are in between the musical and psychological language. In the intermediary words, the analogy will be established. In other words, the intermediary language is the analogous language.

I will use an improvisation of a case that will be described in more detail in Chapter Nine (see Smeijsters & Van den Hurk, 1999). In this case, near the end of therapy the client's musical form had changed. I will focus on the critical episodes in one particular session (Session 22).

The client played the piano on the right side (high-tone register); the music therapist played on the left (low-tone register). Table 7.1, from top to bottom, gives the process in time. The top category gives the musical form; the middle category gives the intermediary words (the analogous language); and the words used for the last category come from analytical developmental psychology and psychotherapy (the psychological language).

Because the intermediary language is an in-between one, the concepts in the middle category have musical and psychological meaning at the same time. So, these concepts on the one hand can be linked to the processes of music, and on the other can be linked to the psychological concepts.

This table should not be interpreted as a universal theory in which the concepts have been linked to each other once and for all. On the contrary, it is a local theory that is credible for this particular client. Keep in mind that this credibility has been researched through a qualitative research study in which transcripts of videotapes and self-reports from the client and the music therapist have been analyzed by means of repeated analysis, member checking, peer debriefing, and triangulation (multiple sources, research techniques, and theories). What I want to show is the possibility of developing an intermediary language in between the musical and psychological language (*Table 7.1*).

Table 7.1

*Music Therapy Helping to Work Through Grief and Finding a Personal Identity (Session 22)**

Section One

- Musical forms: MT plays melody, client plays accompaniment
- Intermediary language**: integrating
- Psychological forms**: individuation and socialization

Section Two

- Musical forms: MT plays crescendo/decrescendo, dotted rhythm; client imitates dynamics and rhythm
- Intermediary language: following
- Psychological form: identification

Section Three

- Musical forms: both MT and client play synchronous phrases
- Intermediary language: fusing
- Psychological form: symbiosis

Section Four

- Musical forms: MT plays rhythm, client plays personal rhythm that fits into the rhythm of the MT
- Intermediary language: integrating
- Psychological forms: individuation and socialization

Section Five

- Musical forms: Both MT and client play sforzati together, finish together, synchronous rhythm
- Intermediary language: fusing
- Psychological form: symbiosis

Section Six

- Musical forms: MT sings, client joins singing with personal motifs
- Intermediary language: integrating
- Psychological forms: individuation and socialization

Section Seven

- Musical forms: Both MT and client play sforzati together, rests, and finish together
- Intermediary language: fusing
- Psychological form: symbiosis

Section Eight

- Musical forms: MT sings, client imitates melody with her voice
- Intermediary language: following
- Psychological form: identification

Section Nine

- Musical forms: Both MT and client play rhythmic swing together, finish together, chords synchronously
- Intermediary language: fusing
- Psychological form: symbiosis

Section Ten

- Musical forms: client sings previous melody of MT with variations
- Intermediary language: making variations
- Psychological form: development of Self

Section Eleven

- Musical forms: MT and client play sforzati together, rests synchronously
- Intermediary language: fusing
- Psychological form: symbiosis

Section Twelve

- Musical forms: MT plays rhythmic legato, client plays atmospheric melody

- Intermediary language: fusing
- Psychological form: symbiosis

Section Thirteen

- Musical forms: both MT and client play pastoral musical dialogue
- Intermediary language: dialoguing
- Psychological form: attunement

Section Fourteen

- Musical forms: MT plays strong figure, client plays melody in the background
- Intermediary language: integrating
- Psychological form: individuation and socialization

Section Fifteen

- Musical forms: both MT and client decrescendo together
- Intermediary language: fusing
- Psychological form: symbiosis

Section Sixteen

- Musical forms: MT plays motif in the bass, client plays soft melting tones
- Intermediary language: fusing
- Psychological form: symbiosis

Section Seventeen

- Musical forms: MT plays rhythmic background, client plays melodic figure
- Intermediary language: integrating
- Psychological forms: individuation and socialization

*Smeijsters & Van den Hurk, 1999.
**Intermediary language and psychological forms describe the client's behaviors/experiences (not the music therapist's). For the intermediary language, I used concepts from Bruscia's integration profile, variability profile, and autonomy profile (Bruscia, 1987).

This improvisation shows that the client in the music in Session 22 was able to fuse, follow, and integrate; to make variations; and to dialogue. These musical forms sound the ability of the client to individualize and socialize. When she started music therapy, she had a low feeling of identity, which since her childhood she had compensated for by not being close to other persons and acting as a tough person, which resulted in rigid behavior. She was unable to go into symbiosis, and to have identification with another person. There was a lack of Self-development within the social contact, a lack of balance between individuation and socialization, and a lack of attunement.

This improvisation shows that the client improved strongly. On the one hand, by playing her own musical motifs, she discovered and developed her personal musical identity, and by this she distinguished herself from the music therapist. On the other hand, her personal musical expressions were part of a shared musical space. The dynamics were developed synchronously, the rhythms were complementary, and there was an exact timing of phrases between the music therapist and the client. The client imitated rhythmic and melodic motifs of the music therapist, but also initiated sounds herself. Sometimes she played a musical background for the music therapist's melodic figure; at other times, she played a melodic figure on the music therapist's ground. These musical forms illustrate how the social and the individual were integrated.

Table 7.1 shows that it is possible to use words, which are in between and are able to bridge the distance between the musical and psychological language. The concepts in the middle category are musical/psychological at the same time. For instance, *following* can be used as a purely musical concept in saying that one imitates a melodic or rhythmic motif and so on. However, following can also be used as a psychological concept, when it refers to one person behaving like somebody else. When taking this further, following can be connected to the process of *identification*. In identification, somebody identifies himself with somebody else, taking over thoughts, feelings, and behaviors to build his identity. When there is a lack of identity, to be like somebody else gives a feeling of identity. When growing up, children find an identity by identifying with their parents, just as teenagers identify with their peers, their musical subgroups, and stars from pop culture.

At some phase of development, this process of identification is passed and the person is able to develop his own authentic and independent identity. Thus, after adolescence the "hired" identity gradually will be replaced by an authentic personal identity. Identification is a normal phase in the process of individuation. However, if there is a fixation, a person will always need another person to get a feeling of identity. It can also be the case that a person fills his lack of identity by overcompensating. In the latter case, because of the lack of identity, the person fears the other's identity, is unable to identify with someone else, and develops tough, autonomous, eccentric, and asocial characteristics, which really do not belong to him. By doing this, he gets a feeling of identity (which is not a real identity). In both cases, the fixation of identification and the overcompensation, there is a false identity. If the person is healthy, there is a balance between the individual and the social. There is a feeling of personal identity, which means that the person does not need identification anymore, nor its counterpart, the asocial counteridentity. He can go into relationships without losing himself. The process of *individuation* in the musical improvisation is sounded in the balance of fusing, following, and integrating.

When constructing the intermediary language, it is important that *following* in the music by the client is *experienced* as identification. The credibility of the local theory depends on the process of member checking, which is part of the therapeutic process itself and part of naturalistic/constructivist inquiry.

EPILOGUE: REDEFINING ANALOGY

Finally, I would like to repeat that fundamental to analogy is that musical processes sound psychological processes, and that changing psychological processes by means of musical processes is therapeutic.

He who identifies the psychological and musical process too absolutely might suggest that the aesthetic forms of music are therapeutic. However, aesthetic forms have their own rules, which do not automatically have psychological significance. Thus, if a client's aesthetic form improves, this does not prove that he is cured. To be sure that it is a psychological improvement, we need to ask which psychological change is sounded in this musical change, and whether this change sounds a psychological change the client needs to become more healthy. What I am saying is that making music is not therapeutic anyway. We need to describe the musical process as a psychological process, and then decide which musical process is indicated according to the client's psychological needs.

I am opposed to the statement that "music therapists are artists," because it suggests that the aesthetic forms are therapeutic. Music therapists are not musicians who listen to and follow the aesthetic rules of music; they are therapists who listen to and follow the psychological processes that are sounded in music. As Pavlicevic puts it: "... the tempo of the client's musical utterances will elicit a response from the music therapist that relates to the client's tempo—not because this is musically appropriate, but rather, because it is personally and relationally appropriate" (Pavlicevic, 2000, p. 276). For the client, the big issue is that he experiences that his forms of feeling are sounded in the music, and that by changing his music he is changing his forms of feeling.

Last but not least, the theory of analogy is never finished. It should be redefined all the time, by means of triangulation with new clinical cases, and concepts from psychological and musical theories.

Chapter Eight

THE ANALOGY OF MUSICAL INTERACTION AND THE DEVELOPMENT OF AN INDEPENDENT SELF

INTRODUCTION

In this chapter, the analogy between interpersonal processes and music improvisation will be explored. Musical form in itself can be like psychosocial processes in a nonsymbolic way, which means that there is a direct and immediate similarity.

The development of musical form has not been accidental, or was not just a process of music theory thinking, but reflects man's search for analogies of his psychological processes. Musical forms have been used for centuries because on an unconscious level they sound psychological processes. If musical forms are completely disconnected from these psychological processes, they lose their meaning. Let me say it in another way: We like what is alike. As Stern (1985) tells us, this similarity is no unimodal "imitation." There is similarity, but it is there in another dimension. We will go into this further later on.

What we should not forget also is that during history, mankind develops and psychological processes change. People from our century who are driving their cars, watching TV, and communicating through the Internet are different from people living in previous centuries. I am not saying that emotions are different. But the different lifestyle has led to changes in the tempo, rhythm, and dynamics of life: the "vitality affects" of life. Because these aspects of life have changed, musical forms have changed with them. But this does not change the basic proposition that the musical form sounds in a way analogous to the psychological process. There are no universal laws of musical form, because "the times, they are a-changing." On the other hand, musical forms cannot be at random because they need to be connected to psychological processes.

What I want to show to you in the following pages is that there is this analogy between musical form and psychological process. First, I will give one example to make clear my way of reasoning.

Take Gestalt psychology, which originally was a psychology of perception. The Gestalt psychologists found that there are Gestalt laws such as "figure-background," "nearness," "similarity," "good continuation," and "closing."

These laws are experienced during visual and auditory perception.

Now let us have a closer look at the Gestalt law of closing. When listening to a piece of music, human beings expect that there will be some sort of finish. There can be a note with long duration, a pause, or a harmonic cadence. All kinds of closings have been used in music.

During music history, composers experimented a lot with how to finish. This is because they wanted to increase tension. In music history, there is a process of tension increase, which shows us that people not only long for endings and tension release, but also for variations in endings and tension increase. Even when there is a need for variation (tension), there is still the longing for the closing that brings it to an end.

Listeners adjust to variations with the result that tension decreases. When for the first time a "Trugschluß" (chord progression V-VI) was used, listeners were aroused because this was different from a normal ending (V-I). After some time, they changed expectations and learned that a Trugschluß was one of the possibilities for ending. This tension decrease forced the composer to establish new variations to evoke new tensions. Musical forms on the one hand include endings, and on the other hand, variations, because human beings need variations and tension increases, too. Because composers used these laws—even before Gestalt psychologists defined them—listening to music became an important part of humans' psychological life.

There is much more to say about these laws. They are not only laws of perception, they are laws of experience. Human beings are not longing just for a closing of sounds; they also have a wish to close experiences of any kind. For instance, grieving after a beloved one has died or after a person has become handicapped implies the need to come to an end with previous life expectations. This life event is about "closing," not in visual or auditory perception, but in a psychological dimension of life. Previous experiences need to be closed before new experiences can be initiated.

As we saw before, in music there are many possibilities to finish a musical process. When a music therapist with his client explores how to finish an improvisation, this is as if they are exploring how to come to an end in a more general way. Musical ending can be experienced as finishing a life event. This experience can be unconscious or conscious; it can become verbally processed or not.

In previous chapters, I defined analogy and its connection to vitality affects. In the upcoming sections, I go deeper into the ways of interaction as described by Stern and then show how these ways of interaction come to sound in music therapy.

THEME AND VARIATION BETWEEN MOTHER AND CHILD

Stern (1985, 1994, 1995) describes how the infant between 2 and 7 months develops a *core Self*. As has been described in Chapter Six, having a sense of a core Self means that there is: *self-agency* (the sense of authorship of one's own actions), *self-coherence* (having a sense of being a nonfragmented physical whole), *self-affectivity* (experiencing patterned inner qualities of feeling that belong with other experiences of Self), and *self-history* (having a sense of a continuity with one's past).

Between these 2 and 6 months, the infant is socially oriented. Stern explored how in this social period interactions are shaped so that a core Self and a core other can develop. This is of interest to a therapist because it is by means of interactions that the core Self develops. In therapy, the relationship and resulting interactions are important change agents.

In Stern's line of reasoning, there are three processes that take place: the caregiver's exaggerated behaviors to get the attention of the infant, the infant perceiving in these behaviors the invariants that reflect the core other, and, finally, the infant distinguishing the core Self from the core other.

The first process, the caregiver's behaviors to get attention, is described as a "theme and variation" format. Stern gives several examples.

"Hello ... Hellooo ... Helllooooo!"

Stern calls this a regular process in time with limited but constant variability. Let us go further into this. In this example, the onset of the stimuli is well timed because the pauses between the words are the same. When a word has finished, you know exactly that after the same time duration a new word will come. At the end of each word, there is no doubt about when the new word will begin. One could say that the tempo from the last "o" to the next "h" is stable.

But the word that follows does not have the same duration as the previous one. This variation brings excitement, and you try to predict how it will be. After some time, you find out that the duration of the words increases at a constant rate. Together with the constant pauses, it gives you a feeling of predictability. There is some sort of a mathematical series in it. Graphically:

***** ___ ******* ___ **********

This time scheme makes anticipation possible although the duration of the words expands. There is not a rigid division of time as in a musical meter; therefore anticipation is exciting, but there is a "rule" in it, which can be discovered.

If there were a rigid fixation in time, then, for the baby it would be boring. Now that there are fluctuations that are predictable, the baby is stimulated to discover the time plan. Discovering the time plan of the partner stimulates the baby to give attention to the partner and makes it possible to predict the partner's sequence and take part in an exciting, playful interaction.

There are several possibilities to include variations. In "Hello ... Hellooo ... Hellloooo!" the pauses were constant and the duration of the words changed. When the words stay the same but the pauses are varied, you get: "Hello, Honey ... Hello, Honey ...... Hello, Honey ....". Graphically:

***** ***** __ ***** ***** __ __ ***** ***** __ __ __

Even when the duration of the pauses and the duration of the words is constant, you can imagine how the mother, by changing the pitch, timbre, and dynamics of the words, can include variation. When a mother touches the baby's nose with her nose three times, each time she will dramatically change the tempo and range of her movements and the accompanying sounds (Stern, 1995).

These examples can be linked to Piaget's concept of *conservation* (Piaget, 1970). Conservation originally was introduced by Piaget to describe the ability in the stage of the concrete operations where the child is able to perceive that in a stimulus some aspects stay the same and others have changed. His experiments—such as the one in which water is transferred from a narrow high bottle into a wide low one—have to do with logical reasoning.

We should be careful when making links between theories. First, the link between Piaget's "conservation and variation" and Stern's "theme and variation" must not be made too strict, because Piaget describes children from 7 years on in the stage of concrete operations and Stern describes babies between 2 and 7 months.

Second, there is the question pointed out by Hargreaves (1988), who doubts if what has been called "conservation in music" is the same as Piaget's concept of conservation. In the experiments of Piaget, the child was able to see the transformations of the objects. The objects also could be retransformed to the original shape. In music, the child listens to two distinct excerpts (the theme and its varied repetition). It is not possible to make visible the process of transition.

Although Piaget's theory has been criticized a lot, I want to use the concept of conservation and variation in this context, and define it as "same and different." One of the perspectives that can be taken into account from a psychological point of view when thinking about "theme and variation" is the conceptual category of "conservation and variation," which in my opinion is a more general category.

Conservation and variation play a role in the perception of the baby. The baby is not able to reason about it, but reacts to it by giving attention to it or turning away from it. The balance of conservation and variation is the psychological essence of the musical form called "theme and variation." It gives continuity in experience and at the same time is challenging.

Stern refers to Piaget when saying that the baby wants to be stimulated and wants to engage actively by making comparisons between new and old stimuli. The baby cannot tell us what he is doing and is not conscious about it, but if the baby's reactions are different when there are different balances of conservation and variation, then we may conclude that the baby notices it. When there is only repetition, when things stay the same, then the baby gets bored. When there is no conservation at all, when all aspects change at the same time, then there is an overload of information. The baby does not "understand" this and will avoid the stimulus. To hold the attention of the baby, there must be a balance of resemblance and contrast. Let us go into some other examples of the mother's interaction with the baby.

"Watcha Doing, Honey?"

Another example is the following:

> Hey, honey … Yeah, honey … Hi, honey …
> Watcha doing, honey? … Yeah, whatcha doing? …
> What are ya doing? … what are ya doing there? … ya doing nothing?
> (Stern, 1985, p. 73; underlined by Stern)

If we transform this example into musical form, it becomes this:

> a-b … a'-b … a''-b …
> c-b … a'-c …
> d-c' … d-c'-e … c'-f

We see several types of variations:

1) A variation of sound: a / a' / a'' (hey / yeah / hi)
2) Different combinations: a-b / c-b (hey, honey / watcha doing, honey?)
3) Different sequences: c-b / a'-c (watcha doing, honey? / yeah, watcha doing?); d-c' / c'-f (what are ya doing? / ya doing nothing?)
4) Shortening: c / c' (whatcha doing? / ya doing?)
5) Extension: d-c' / d-c'-e (what are ya doing? / what are ya doing there?)

These variations together give the impression that there is variation in conservation. Composers of music use these procedures when building musical forms. Astonishingly, mothers (and fathers as well) are able to do this without training and reflection, but by means of active listening to the baby. Caregivers who do not have the competence to listen and look at the baby's reaction and to immediately adjust their pattern of conservation and variation cannot give the baby satisfying experiences that lead to a healthy interaction and development of Self.

"I'm Gonna Get You"

Stern gives further examples. For example, the body-touching game that includes "I'm gonna get you" when the mother walks with her fingers on the infant's torso.

> "I' m g o n n a g e t y o u"
> "I' m g o n n a g e t y o u"
> "I'm gonna get you"

The game ends after the final "I'm gonna get you" and a tickling of the child in the neck or on the chin. In this example, the words stay the same. What changes is the tempo (from slow to fast), the accompanying melodic line of the words, and the rhythm and distance travelled of the fingers on the child's body.

At a later stage of development, when the child is older and able to walk, parents play this game by starting from a distance, walking gradually faster into the child's direction, and in the final run taking the child in the arms. At the end, there always is a release of tension, and laughter.

In both cases, the finger tickling and walking from a distance, the situation for the child is very exciting because synchronously to a speeding up of tempo in the words, and thus a shortening of phrasing in time, the distance in space that is bridged over increases. In a shorter time, a longer distance is passed through.

Another way to play this game is the other way around:

> "I'm gonna get you"
> "I' m g o n n a g e t y o u"
> "I' m g o n n a g e t y o u"
> (Stern 1994, p. 114)

Before going into the conservation and variation in music and music therapy, let me draw some conclusions.

A first important conclusion that can be drawn from these examples is that when, as Stern is telling us, the core Self precedes merging, then the first phase in therapy should be establishing conservation and variation in interaction, and not, as Mahler (1975) suggests, symbiosis.

A second conclusion is about the way Stern describes how self-invariants develop. If in music therapy developing an "organized sense of Self" is a goal, then music therapists should develop musical actions whereby the client feels his personal will to act, feels himself being an actor, experiences that his action causes effects, and so on.

A third point is Stern's remark that only major psychosis shows a significant absence of any of the core Self senses. Psychotic patients suffer from derealization and delusions (no agency), depersonalization, incoherent thinking and fusion (no coherence), flattened affects (no affectivity), fugue and dissociation (no continuity). We might conclude that the developmental stage of the core Self can be used as a goal when working with psychotic patients. However, clinical practice shows that the principle of conservation and variation can be used in the treatment of many other disturbances and handicaps.

CONSERVATION AND VARIATION IN MUSIC AND MUSIC THERAPY

A close analogy to the stage of interaction in which the core Self develops is the conservation and variation in music therapy. Then there is an exchange that is not pre-established but developing in the here-and-now moment.

In the following section, I will first look into the musical phenomenon from a psychological point of view, and explore how conservation and variation can be established. Then I will focus on the possibilities of conservation and variation in music therapy interaction.

Conservation and Variation in Music

Before going into several types of "conservation and variation," let me summarize several aspects:

- "Conservation and variation" means that parts of an object are kept stable, whereas other parts change. "Theme and variation" are an example of "conservation and variation," because something is conserved and something else is changing.
- In the baby, there is some perceptual ability to "understand" conservation and variation.

- "Conservation and variation," in a right mix, secure that the attention of the baby will be maintained. When the mother does not use variations, the baby after some time will get bored; when the changes are too enormous, the baby becomes frightened.
- From a certain stage of development, the child is able to understand and to point out, after a transformation of an object, what is equal and what is different.

In this part, I will concentrate on conservation and variation in musical processes in time. In the section on music therapy, I will distinguish between synchronously and sequenced conservation and variation in music therapy interaction.

CONSERVATION AND VARIATION IN MUSIC IN TIME. In conservation and variation in music in time, there is a theme or musical part which, when repeated, becomes varied. From a musical point of view, this conservation and variation can be divided in two broad categories. In a melodic theme and variation, a melodic basic structure is kept the same, but melodic ornaments and figures are added that obscure the original melodic line. This conservation and variation take place within the *same parameter*. Another type of conservation and variation would be a theme and variation where the melody is kept intact but there are changes in *accompanying parameters*—for example, when rhythm and/or harmony change.

Types of conservation have been researched in the developmental psychology of music: (Pflederer, 1964, 1967), Pflederer and Sechrest (1968), Rider (1977, 1981), and Serafine (1980).

In the next section, I will give examples of several possibilities within the two categories.

CONSERVATION AND VARIATION WITHIN THE SAME PARAMETER. There is conservation and variation in the same parameter when the listener, for instance, "knows" that:

- When a *melody* is ornamented, there is still the same basic melodic line in it
- When a *rhythm* becomes more differentiated, there are still the same rhythmic cornerstones in it
- When a *chord* is extended with a single tone (for example, a fourth or a sixth), there is still the same chord building

However, as Gestalt psychology shows, one single element can change the whole impression. For instance, the septime changes the whole impression of the chord. Thus, whether the listener hears the basic structure or gets a completely different impression depends on the type of variation.

CONSERVATION AND VARIATION BETWEEN DIFFERENT PARAMETERS. There are many examples of conservation and variation between musical parameters. Let me give you some examples:

- When there is a change of rhythm and the meter is kept stable
- When there is a change of rhythm and the melody is kept stable
- When there is a change of tempo and the melody is kept stable
- When there is a change of dynamics and other parameters are kept stable
- When there is a change of instrument and the melody is kept stable
- When there is a change of instrument and the rhythm is kept stable
- When there is a change of duration (e.g., augmentation or diminuation) and the melody is kept stable
- When there is a change of intervals and the contour is kept stable
- When there is a change of key (pitch)
- When there is a change from major to minor
- When there is a change of harmony and the melody is kept stable

It is possible to change more than one parameter at the time (for example, speed and dynamics).

What is important for music therapy is to explore which changes are close to conservation and which are close to variation. I think that some of these options give the impression of change, whereas others do not (as has been said before on Gestalt psychology). For their use in music therapy, this is very important.

Conservation and Variation in Same and Different Parameters in Music Therapy: Sequential and Synchronous

In the previous part, there has been made a distinction between conservation and variation within the same and between different parameters. Both categories refer to sequences in time, which means that there first is the exhibition of a theme and then variations follow in the same or another parameter.

In music therapy, as in the mother-child interaction, another type of conservation and variation is possible because mother and child, music therapist and client, act synchronously, at the same time. Two categories can be added, then: the synchronous conservation and variation within the same parameter, and the synchronous conservation and variation between different parameters.

Bruscia (1987), in his 64 clinical techniques of improvisational music therapy, described sequential and synchronous types of conservation and variation in music therapy. One of Bruscia's techniques, called *imitating,* brings us to an important discussion. "Imitating" is described as:

> "Echoing or reproducing a client's response after the response has been completed." (Bruscia, 1987, p. 535)

For instance, a client plays a melodic motif and the music therapist repeats the motif after the client has stopped. The technique is within the same musical parameter (melody), and there is no variation. The discussion this technique evokes is whether it can be a technique of empathy.

Stern (1995) gives an example of how the mother reacts empathically. When the baby's face expression reflects an inner feeling of delight, the mother might imitate this facial expression and thus react in the same modus (visual). Stern argues that in this case the baby sees only that the mother does the same he does. He just sees a mirror, but cannot be sure that there is a Self inside this mirror. But when the mother reacts in another modus (sound) and for example says "YeeeEEEEsss," the pitch (up and down), the duration (augmentation), and the dynamics (crescendo and decrescendo) of her words reflect the baby's facial expression and feeling. By this cross-modal answer, according to Stern, the baby knows that there is somebody outside who is able to transform his feeling and facial expression into words and sounds.

In Stern's example, the modus changes from vision to sound, but some parameters are the same. For instance, the duration of the smile (which is an expression of the child's feeling) is the same as the duration of the sound, the increase and decrease of intensity of the smile is the same as the crescendo and decrescendo of the sound, and so on.

Stern concludes that because of the "analogy" in the mother's answer (Stern, 1995, p. 113), empathy becomes possible. "Analogy" means using a different modus with the same parameters. A second conclusion would be that "imitating" is less important than responding by conservation and variation. According to Stern, during conservation and variation, your partner feels that there is an independent human being who is different but feels the same. It is the conservation and variation that tells you that there is a core other, which is distinguished from the core Self but feels the same. Here also, Stern withdraws from the idea of symbioses.

When "empathy" needs some type of variation—reacting in a different modus, within the same modus in a different parameter, or by variation in the same parameter—then "imitating" as described by Bruscia cannot be a genuine technique of empathy. In "imitating," the music therapist reproduces the client's response in the same modus, the same parameter, without variation.

In music therapy, the music therapist and client—whether using instruments or voice—are communicating in the same modus (music). There is no cross-modality; therefore, the music therapist should be aware that "imitating" might hinder the communication of empathy. When the music therapist cannot "attune" to the client in another modus, the development of variations within the same parameter or between different parameters will be necessary.

CONSERVATION AND VARIATION IN THE SAME PARAMETER IN MUSIC THERAPY, AFTER THE CLIENT'S RESPONSE HAS BEEN COMPLETED: RHYTHMIC DIMINUTION AND AUGMENTATION IN MUSIC THERAPY. Diminution and augmentation are variations in the parameter of rhythm. In diminution, the durations of tones are shortened. For instance, crotchets are changed into quavers, and then into semiquavers. The other way around is called "augmentation."

Diminution enhances the tempo because when the durations are shortened, the impulses will come more quickly. Let me give you one example where this change of tempo is used to establish a relaxed and joyful atmosphere.

When clients are sitting in a circle, they can become invited to pass through to their neighbor a single tone or rhythmic motif that becomes shortened each time the tone has gone around the complete circle. The members of the group need to be fully aware because the timing changes quickly. As a result of this, there will be members who make "mistakes" by reacting too early or too late. Because everybody knows that this is what it is all about in this game, when "mistakes" are made, there is laughter and a short stop, which releases tension. Making "mistakes" in this game, where mistakes are planned as part of it, show the client that everybody makes mistakes, that making mistakes is no threat, and that he need not worry about it. It is a musical game where relaxation is reached by tension enhancement and subsequent tension release.

Ornamenting types of rhythmical diminution can be used in music therapy also. Ornamenting means putting tones with short duration in between the original tones. It can be used in cases where clients—for instance, autistics—are resistant to variation. By gradually adding new tones and at the same time keeping intact the original structure, the music therapist intends to bring clients to the acceptance of newness.

The music therapist can use augmentation as a technique for "redirecting" (Bruscia, 1987). He can slow down the musical process to calm the client's expression.

CONSERVATION AND VARIATION IN THE SAME PARAMETER IN MUSIC THERAPY, AFTER THE CLIENT'S RESPONSE HAS BEEN COMPLETED: RHYTHMIC, MELODIC, AND TIMBRE VARIATION IN MUSIC THERAPY. Rhythmic, melodic, or timbre variations within the same parameter after the client's response have been completed can occur, for instance, when a client sings or plays one single tone duration and the music therapist reacts to it by structuring it rhythmically, or when the music therapist reacts by making melodic variations in the client's melodic motif, or when the music therapist varies the timbre of the voice or instrument.

CONSERVATION AND VARIATION BETWEEN DIFFERENT PARAMETERS IN MUSIC THERAPY AFTER THE CLIENT'S RESPONSE HAS BEEN COMPLETED. As we described before, when there is conservation and variation between different parameters, a musical excerpt is repeated, and some parameters are imitated exactly, whereas other parameters change. The examples in a previous part show that each parameter (tempo, rhythm, and so on) can be "conserved" and combined with variations in other parameters.

When can it be used in music therapy? There may be the same intention of the mother trying to hold the attention of the baby. However, in music therapy there is another important goal. Several client groups that are treated by music therapists—for example, the mentally handicapped, the autistic, and the schizophrenic—for different reasons need a lot of repetition and are unable to accept variations easily. There is no need for variation to stay aware—as with the baby—but there is a need for repetition and strong predictability, so that their personal frame of reference will not be disrupted too much. Another way of looking at this is to say that their balance of conservation and variation differs. These clients need more conservation and less variation.

The intention of the music therapist is to change this balance and to stimulate them to accept variations. Acceptance of variations means that they can be more open to and able to cope with their outer world, which is full of variations. By means of different levels of conservation and variation in music, this openness can be approached.

SYNCHRONOUS CONSERVATION AND VARIATION BETWEEN DIFFERENT PARAMETERS. Bruscia (1987) described the "pacing" technique of empathy as follows:

> "Matching the client's energy level (i.e., intensity and speed)" (Bruscia, 1987, p. 535).

Pacing occurs when, for instance, the music therapist and the client at the same time play crescendo, decrescendo, loud, soft, accelerando, ritardando, slow, or fast. In essence, "pacing" means that the music therapist adapts to the client's dynamics and tempo.

The "pacing" technique is especially interesting because "intensity" and "speed" are very close to what Stern has called "vitality affects." Just remember his definition: "... vitality affects are kinetic qualities of feelings such as surging, fading away, fleeting, explosive, crescendo, decrescendo, bursting, drawn out ..." (Stern, 1985, p. 54). Some of these changes are characterized by changes in *intensity* (tending to explode, increasing volume, decreasing volume) and *tempo* (passing rapidly, appearing suddenly). Intensity and speed are both basic characteristics of vitality affects. When a client is changing intensity and speed, there is a change in his vitality affects. Using the "pacing" technique—matching the client's intensity and speed—means matching the client's vitality affects.

When "pacing," the music therapist can use "conservation and variation" when he matches the client's dynamics and tempo, but at the same time use melodies, rhythms, and harmonies that differ from the client's melodies, rhythms, and harmonies. Then there is conservation (same) in the parameters of dynamics and tempo and variation in other parameters (different). Because of this, on the one hand the client is able to be aware of someone else who matches the intensity and speed of his own vitality affects, but also feels that there is another independent Self with a unique musical identity.

SYNCHRONOUS CONSERVATION AND VARIATION BETWEEN DIFFERENT MODI. In music therapy, working in different modi is possible—for example, when the music therapist gives a musical answer or chooses a piece of music that corresponds to what he thinks the client is experiencing or expressing nonverbally. The music therapist transforms experiences into music. "Reflecting," as described by Bruscia (1987, p. 535), is "...matching the moods, attitudes, and feelings exhibited by the client" and an example of this. This can be done in receptive as well as active music therapy.

When a client is not making sounds himself, then this is an opportunity for the music therapist to react in the music, which is a modus different from the client's modus of expression. There are many examples of this, but I will focus on two, one from the Nordoff-Robbins school of music and one from the German music therapist Karin Schumacher.

In *Creative Music Therapy* (1977), Nordoff and Robbins describe two techniques where cross-modality is used. The first one has been called "creating a musical-emotional environment"; the second, "making music according the movements of a musically nonactive child." In the first technique, the music therapist tries to create music that reflects the mood of the child. This is much more difficult than the second technique, because in the first technique the music therapist by means of empathy needs to explore the child's mood. This point illustrates that empathy has two aspects: One is the therapist's inner feeling of how the client is feeling, while the second aspect is communicative, showing the client that the music therapist is feeling how the client is feeling.

In the second technique, this is different and less difficult because the client is behaving. This behavior corresponds to an inner mood that should be empathically felt by the therapist too, but because of the observable behaving of the client, it is much easier to adjust to the client. The behavior of the client helps the music therapist to choose the empathic musical ingredients by adjusting his musical parameters to the client's movement behavior.

In the first technique, "creating a musical-emotional environment," the music sounds as the vitality affects of the mood. In the second technique, "making music according the movements of a musically nonactive child," every rhythmic body movement modus—jumping, swinging, making movements with the hand and fingers—is accompanied by the auditory modus.

Schumacher (1994, 1999), who based her work with autistic children on Stern's psychology, developed techniques of acceptance such as:

- *Music in the environment, creating nearness and distance*: The music therapist tries to understand the psychological condition of the child and makes music that attunes to it. There is no need for the child to play; the music therapist does not invite the child and somehow plays for herself. By doing this, she creates an atmosphere that communicates the acceptance of the child's condition.
- *Creating resonance, music for the child*: The music therapist contains in her music the breath movement of an inactive child or the (stereotyped) body movements and verbal sounds of an active child. The music therapist moves herself, uses musical sounds and "situation songs" in which the words describe how the child presents himself to the music therapist by his movement and his actions.
- *Creating a coordinated evocative climate, music coming from the child*: The child still is musically inactive. The music therapist creates "intermodal connections" (Schumacher), and puts the inner affect of the child into sound and makes the child experience "I hear what I sense." Essential to this technique is, as Schumacher puts forward, the development of the client's inter-affectivity, when two persons experience the same affect. It is part of the development of the intersubjective Self .

As in the examples from Nordoff and Robbins, these examples from Schumacher show that there is synchronous conservation and variation between different modi.

The Case of Edward: Sequential Conservation and Variation

The "classical" case of Edward, by Paul Nordoff and Clive Robbins (1977), is a famous case that illustrates the possibilities of musical communication. In her analysis of this same case Rolvsjord (1998) refers to Kristeva, who describes the semiotic and symbolic aspects of a text. Semiotic aspects are formed by the musical parameters (rhythm, intonations, timbre, dynamics, and so on). Semiotic expressions have emotional meaning and can be linked to vitality affects and thus to analogy. The case of Edward gives us an impressive example of semiotic expression. Rolsjord follows Kristeva when saying that also in the musical communication the semiotic and symbolic both are present. Symbolic is understood as a set of conventions and rules, which organize music as genre (for instance, western traditional art music).

However, I think that verbal language needs more conventions and rules than does music. A music therapist, in his interaction with the client, can free himself from many traditional musical rules. The (classical) Nordoff and Robbins method of music therapy has been more rules-based and thus more symbolic in Kristeva's sense. Edward's semiotic expression gets part of the symbolic expression that is offered to him by Paul Nordoff and Clive Robbins. Within this symbolic form, Edward's expression can be "understood."

What is very impressive in the case of Edward, from my point of view, is that it illustrates conservation and variation in music therapy very well. The client as well as the music therapist introduces rhythmic, melodic, and timbre variations. As a result of this, a really varied communication develops.

In Session Nine, there is an exchange between Edward and Paul Nordoff, which I call "circular imitation, initiation, and variation" *(Table 8.1).*

Table 8.1

Circular Imitation, Initiation,
and Variation in the Case of Edward
(Session Nine)

Paul Nordoff (at the piano)	Edward
"good morning"(repeated)	
	"ojeoi … ojeoi"
	"… **ello"** (repeated in interaction)
"hello" (repeated in interaction)	
"hi" (repeated in interaction)	
	"hi" (repeated in interaction)
"hello" (repeated in interaction)	
	"… ello" (repeated in interaction)
	"i-i-i-i-i" (descending)

"hello" (repeated in interaction)	
	"… ello" (repeated in interaction)
	"… eh … eh"
"hello" (repeated in interaction)	
	"iiiii-iiiii" (repeated in interaction)
	"he-he" (descending)
"hoah-hoah" (descending)	
"hello"	
	"… ello" (repeated)
"hello Edward"	
	"i-i-i" (ascending; repeated in interaction)
"i-i-i" (ascending; repeated in interaction)	
	"… ello"
"hello"	
"i-i-i"	
	"i-i-i"
"hello"	
"i-i-i" (repeated in interaction)	
	"i-i-i" (repeated in interaction)
	"i-a-a" (repeated in interaction)
"i-a-a" (repeated in interaction)	
	"ah-ah"
"ah-ah"	
"hello" (repeated in interaction)	
	"… ello" (repeated in interaction)
"Edward" (repeated in interaction)	
	"… eh-eh" (repeated in interaction)
"Edward"	
"i-i-i"	
"Uncle Paul" (Clive Robbins)	
	"i-i-i"
"i-i-i" (ascending sequence; repeated in interaction)	
	"i-i-i" (ascending sequence; repeated in interaction)
"hello"	
"i-i-i"	

	"... aaaahhh"
"ba-ba-ba"	
	"eh-eh-eh-eh"
"ah-ah-ah-ah"	
	"uh-uh-uh-uh"
"ah-ah-ah-ah"	
	"eh-eh-eh-ah"
"ah-ah-ah-ah"	
	"ah-ah-ah-ah"
"ah-ah-ah-ah"	
	"oh-oh-oh-oh"
"oh-oh-oh-oh-oh-oh-oh"	
	"oh-oh"
	"eh-eh"
"hello" (repeated)	
"Edward"	
	"oh-oh-oh-oh"
"Edward"	
	"ueh-ueh"
"E-E-Edward"	
"E-E-Edward"	
	"ah-ah-ah-ah-eih"
"E-E-Edward"	
	"ah-ah-ah-ieh"
"E-E-Edward"	
	"ah-ah-ah-ieh"
	glissando
glissando	
"hello" (repeated)	
"good-bye good-bye good-bye"	
	"ah-ah-ah-ah-ah-ah-ah-ah"
"ah-ah-ah-ah-ah-ah"	
"aaaaaaaaaaaaaaaaahhhhhhhhhh"	
	"jjjjoooo"
"jjjjaaaa"	
	"jjjjaaaa"
"nnnnoooo"	
	"nnjjoooo"
"noooo"	
	"i-i-i-i"
"i-i-i-i"	
	"i-i-i-ei"

"Edward"	
"Edward"	
	"ooohhh"
"oh-oh"	
	"oh-oh"
	"oh-oeh"
"good-bye" (repeated in interaction)	
	"good-bye" (repeated in interaction)
"Edward good-bye"	

In Table 8.1, bold signifies Edward taking initiative and Paul Nordoff imitating; underlining signifies Nordoff taking initiative and Edward imitating.

When Edward *initiates* "ello," Nordoff *imitates* "Hello." Then Nordoff takes over and initiates "Hi," and Edward imitates "Hi." When Edward initiates "i-i-i," Nordoff immediately responds by singing "i-i-i." At other times, Nordoff initiates "i-i-i" himself. When Edward initiates "i-i-i-i," again, Nordoff imitates this motif immediately. This process goes on and on and is characterized by its *circularity*. It is a communication of people listening and imitating each other but also offering new elements to each other. Nordoff, when imitating, sometimes *extends* the motif. For example, when Edward sings "oh-oh-oh-oh," Nordoff sings "oh-oh-oh-oh-oh-oh-oh."

Nordoff also puts in *variations*. For instance, when Edward sings "jjjjoooo," Nordoff sings "jjjjaaaa." Edward, in his imitating, makes variations, too. For example, when he answers "eh-eh-eh-eh," "uh-uh-uh-uh," "eh-eh-eh-ah," "ah-ah-ah-ah," "oh-oh-oh-oh."

There are times when there is a *triangle* of initiation, imitation, and variation. When Edward sings "... aaaahhh" (initiates), Nordoff takes the same sound "a" (imitates), makes a rhythmic structure out of it "ba-ba-ba" (varies), and then Edward imitates this rhythmic structure and at the same tame varies the sound and extends the motif when singing "eh-eh-eh-eh." This is followed by Nordoff repeating the sound "a," and imitating the extended motif: "ah-ah-ah-ah." At another occasion, Edward initiates "ooohhh," and Nordoff imitates the sound and at the same time varies its structure by singing "oh-oh." Then Edward imitates this structure with "oh-oh," which is followed by his variation of sound: "oh-oeh." We can conclude that in this interaction there are two processes: a circular process of *imitation and initiation*, and a process of *imitation and variation*.

To develop communication, both aspects seem to be important: Both people should "imitate" the other as well as "initiate" (new) actions themselves. The initiation of new elements also can be described as a "variation of input." Besides this, there is the "variation of answer," when variation occurs within the same parameter. Most significant are the variations in the vocal timbre: for instance, when Edward sings "he-he" and Nordoff answers "hoah-hoah"; or when Nordoff sings "ah-ah-ah-ah" and Edward sings "eh-eh-eh-eh," "uh-uh-uh-uh," "oh-oh-oh-oh"; or when Nordoff sings "E-E-Edward ... E-E-Edward" and Edward answers by singing "ah-ah-ah-ah-eih." Besides variations of timbre, there are melodic variations when they both are exploring glissandi.

There is a lot of imitation in this play. My previous conclusion—based on Stern's findings—that imitation is not a genuine way to communicate empathy, should be reconsidered, then, as follows: Imitation is not a means to communicate empathy on its own; however, in music therapy imitation is part of the triangle of imitation, initiation, and variation.

CONSERVATION AND VARIATION IN LANGUAGE AND MUSIC. Another example shows how the music therapist varies melodic motifs initiated by him. Let's have a look into such a process of variation during a music therapy improvisation (Smeijsters & Van den Berk, 1995, p. 253):

> "In Session 17, the scope of the training was broadened. Whilst the client played a 6/8 rhythm or a march with a dotted rhythm, the music therapist played various melodic fragments in which one or more nuclei were constantly repeated, elaborated and/or varied: f-d, f-d-b, f-d-c-d, f-d-e-c-d, d-f-e-c-d, d-f-e-g-f, a-g-e-f-d, d-g-e-f, d-a-f-g-e-f."

The characters refer to pitches. The underlining shows how the f-d and c-d motifs develop. Categorizing the different developments shows us that the melodic motifs contain:

1) Different linking: d-f-e-c-d / d-f-e-g-f
2) Different sequences: f-d / d-f and d-f-e-g-(f) / (a)-g-e-f-d / d-g-e-f
3) Abbreviation: a-g-e-f-d / d-g-e-f
4) Enlargements: f-d / f-d-b / f-d-c-d and c-d / e-c-d and d-g-e-f / d-a-f-g-e-f

In this particular case, a client with musicogenic epilepsy, who suffered from seizures when playing unpredictable melodies, even though this particular melodic line played by the music therapist was full of variations, suffered no seizures. There were two reasons for this: 1) she was playing a rhythmic ground herself, and 2) the melodic line clearly was characterized by a conservation and variation format.

The caregiver in Stern's examples and the music therapist in this particular case are using techniques of variation. In Stern's example, these techniques are applied to words. The infant does not understand the meaning of the words; he is listening to a combination of sounds, rhythms, and pitches.

However, there are differences between Stern's example and the example from music therapy. Stern calls "honey" and "ya doing" themes because they are repeated. In music, we would call them "cells." In music, a "theme" is a melodic, rhythmic, dynamic, and harmonic extended phrase of several measures, which is closed at the end and forms a Gestalt. It is composed of several cells. In Stern's sense, themes (cells) are stable, repeated, and not varied themselves, whereas the surroundings change. When there is a "theme and variation" in music, the whole theme and the cells within the theme will become varied.

This shows an important difference between possibilities of variation within language and music. To illustrate this further, let me give you an example of cell variation in music. In the example of the music therapy improvisation, melodic cells are:

f-d
c-d
d-f-e-g

The last cell could be identified as a "motif" (a short theme), which by the music therapist is changed inside:

d-f-e-g
g-e-f-d
d-g-e-f

Remember that the characters signify pitches.

If we applied this to the word "honey," then we would have to do it this way:

h-o-n-e-y
y-e-n-o-h
h-y-e-n-o

This makes no sense in language; it is strictly a musical procedure. Although the child cannot understand the word at that time, no parent will vary the word like a musical motif because the word has meaning and by repeating it the meaning slowly can be apprehended by the child. A musical motif can be repeated many times also to stimulate apprehension; however, the possibilities of variation in one musical motif are much more extensive than in language.

The Case of Ingrid: Synchronous Conservation and Variation

Synchronous conservation and variation within the same parameter means that the client's and the music therapist's play in the same parameter is complementary. For example, the music therapist is playing the beat and the client at the same time is playing a rhythm, which fits the beat. Or the music therapist sings a melody and the client sings basic pitches, makes an inversion of the melody, or sings at the same time in a distance of a third, and so on.

In these cases, there is a connection of the client's rhythm to the music therapist's rhythm and of the client's melody to the music therapist's melody. Thus, there is a "conservation" between the rhythms and the melodies because elements are shared, whereas some other elements are different.

Let me give you an example of synchronous conservation and variation in the same parameter taken from the case of Ingrid, a woman 53 years old who, after her husband had died, found it difficult to find a new way of life (Smeijsters & Van den Hurk, 1999; Smeijsters, 1999a).

In the music therapy improvisations, Ingrid again and again tried to play fragments of melodic scales at the piano. She did not succeed in playing them properly, and each time became disappointed and stopped playing. From her verbal comments it became clear that during her life thus far she had held very high standards, which she was not now able to uphold, and which had led to low self-esteem.

During the first sessions, it turned out that when José van den Hurk (the music therapist) accompanied her with a stable rhythmic chord progression, Ingrid was able to free herself from the normative melodic scales. Therefore, Van den Hurk decided to use the "repetition" of the rhythmic harmonic ground as a technique of elicitation (Bruscia, 1987). After some time, Van den Hurk changed her chords by playing successively the single tones of the chords, thus ornamenting by means of melodic/rhythmic diminution. This turned out to be a means to stimulate Ingrid to give way to her feelings by developing a personal melodic theme *(see Table 8.2)*.

Table 8.2

Conservation and Variation in the Case of Ingrid (Session 16)

MT with Piano and Voice	Client Singing
C-major chord	sings soft
quiet, andante	**sings longstanding tones**
sings tones from chord	
moods as in "Rheingold" (Wagner)	
V-IV-I chord progression	***sings sol-si-la-sol***
	sings long tones from chord fundamentals
high-pitched vocal melody	
I-IV-V chord progression	***sings a 3- tone motif***
sings sol-la-sol-fa-re-mi	
makes melodic figures	
plays a dotted rhythm	
sings mi-re-mi-re-do	uses long and short tones
sequences	
sings sol-la-sol-fa-mi-re	
mi-re-do	sings **mi-re-do** with MT
makes a crescendo	
is silent	
	sings dotted rhythm
imitates dotted rhythm	do-**re-mi**-mi-/mi-fa-sol/**mi-do**
completes melody from Cl: **mi-do**/sol-la-sol-fa-mi-**re-mi**/ **re-mi**-re-do	
polyphony develops*	polyphony develops*
sings **mi-fa**-sol-fa-**mi-re-mi-fa-mi-re***	sings **mi-re**-mi-**mi-fa-mi-fa-mi-re***
is silent	makes variations on do-re-mi
accompanies	***solo***
plays melody with right hand*	polyphony*
accompanies	***do-fa-si-sol***
sings melody*	personal rhythm and melody*
crescendo	**crescendo**
sings low tones	
	variations, strong melody
sings melody	***si-do-re-si-do (cadence)***

solo	***long tones***
melody with the right hand*	polyphony*
soft, vocal	***accompanies soft***
rhythmic, crescendo, jazzy, bop*	strong personal melody*
crescendo	**crescendo**
vocal sound effects, **soft**	**soft**, long tones
ritardando, **decrescendo**	**decrescendo**

There are several categories of conservation and variation:

- What is on the left-hand side of the left column and the right-hand side of the right column are very different. There is no interconnection between the music therapist and client.
- What is put in the middle shows some sort of sharing (conservation), and conservation or variation on several levels:
    - Sharing the same tones, durations, rhythms, or dynamics (bold)
    - One person accompanying the other's solo (bold and italic)
    - Both persons finding a personal rhythm and melody (*)

Throughout the improvisation, sharing the same tones, durations, rhythms, or dynamics gave this client—who was insecure in expressing herself—a stable musical ground that gave her a feeling of security.

From the melodic point of view, this improvisation shows how the client developed a personal identity. There was conservation in the same parameter when the music therapist and client shared basic pitches of the chord progression. The music therapist "unfroze" the chord progression by melodic and rhythmic diminution of the chord tones. This was done to stimulate and intensify the client's expression. By means of synchronous variation in the same parameter, the music therapist—while still sharing the same chord fundamentals with the client—developed personal melodic motifs. Throughout the improvisation, there were passages where the music therapist and client accompanied each other. When doing this, one individual came to the musical foreground while the other stayed in the background. Then the client could express her individuality and was backed up by the music therapist. Eventually, in the polyphonic fragments, while still sharing some basic characteristics in the same parameter, the client found an autonomous personal musical identity, while at the same time there was another individual who expressed her own identity.

EPILOGUE: THE ANALOGOUS TRIANGLE

We may conclude that the conservation and variation is part of the interaction between mother and child and between the music therapist and his client. Because of this, there exists an analogy between the development of an independent Self and interaction in music therapy. When improvising with another person, the client experiences personal "invariants" (Stern, 1985) and (re)develops a sense of Self. This makes music therapy appropriate for clients whose sense of Self is disturbed.

Stern (1995) calls the mother's behavior a "choreography" or "orchestration" in which the baby experiences his feelings. There is an analogy between the pattern of interaction and the process of feeling. When the mother is interacting with the baby by means of conservation and variation, she evokes feelings. There is attention, increase of tension, insecurity, a sense of predictability, and, finally, decrease of tension, cognitive processes that are closely linked to emotions. The baby can be happy because of the surprises, because of the predictable process of change, and because of the release.

Musical interaction in music therapy is not just interaction, but a process of feeling by interaction in which feelings are evoked gradually or suddenly, come to a climax, stay for some time, decrease, are evoked again, and so on. In music therapy there is a triangle of music, interaction and the sense of Self.

Chapter Nine

EXAMPLES OF ANALOGY FROM RESEARCH AND CLINICAL PRACTICE

INTRODUCTION

As an illustration of analogy, I will give several examples from case study research and clinical practice. As put forward in previous chapters, analogy means that in diagnostic terms the musical expression of the client has characteristics that are like the characteristics of the client's psychological problems or handicaps. It has been said that the client's problems "sound" in the music. In terms of treatment, analogy means that it is possible to offer the client musical experiences that are similar experiences that lead to more health. In music therapy, the psychological processes of improvement "sound" in the music.

In some other published works, I summarized research that shows a match between DSM-IV items and musical behaviors (Smeijsters, 1995, 1999b, 2000/2003). For instance, clients with a depression play songs on the piano much more slowly than they were used to do (Steinberg & Raith, 1985; Steinberg, Krause, Lerch, & Raith, 1987), and schizophrenic clients are unable to adjust to the music therapist's play (Pavlicevic & Trevarthen, 1989; Pavlicevic, Trevarthen, & Duncan, 1994). As a conclusion, we can say that the experience of time in depression is sounded in the slower tempo of the musical play, and that the isolation of the schizophrenic client is sounded in the lack of contact in the musical interaction.

Examples from my own qualitative single-case research show that a fixed rhythmic pattern can be an analogy of compulsive behavior (Van den Hurk & Smeijsters, 1991) and that the frequent switch between a fast, restless melodic line running up and down and a very tough, stereotyped melodic motif of a few tones can be an analogy of the disturbed communication between the asking child and the rejecting, cool parent (Smeijsters & Van den Hurk, 1993/1994). Suddenly heavy sounds with a rough timbre and bumping harmonies have been described by the client as being abused (Smeijsters & Van den Berk, 1995/1999). The musical behavior of a little girl, playing loud, and behaving against the grain, was an analogy in sound of the way in which the mother felt the child took over her parental power (Smeijsters & Storm, 1997/1998). The inability to find a personal melody was analogous to a felt lack of self-identity (Smeijsters & Van den Hurk, 1999; Smeijsters, 1999a).

In previous chapters, I used some of these research studies to work out aspects of analogy. In this chapter, I will give a more extended description of the analogies that have been developed through these and other research studies. You can see that since 1991 the development of the concept of analogy is reflected in the way the examples have been described. In any case, analogy is different from metaphor and symbol because in analogy the psychological processes are directly sounded in the music. I also will include several examples from other researchers because they give an excellent impression of analogy.

Describing analogies is a matter of many hours of research. Although the descriptions in the following sections are short summaries, in the single-case research I did, the summaries are the result of extensive, thick descriptions of all therapy sessions, which have been the subject of naturalistic inquiry (member checking, peer debriefing, triangulation) and have been content analyzed carefully by means of grounded theory, phenomenology, and hermeneutics.

Although analogy is a general concept, the content of the analogies that are described in this chapter are special, which means that they belong to these clients. One never can say in a universal way that a limited melodic line sounds a feeling of a lack of self-identity, nor that a restricted rhythm sounds compulsive behavior. Of course, there might be some transferability to other cases, but it depends always on the individual case.

One should never forget that the trustworthiness of the hypothesis that musical processes are analogies of the client's vitality affects—and "sound," his psyche—eventually can only be assured by the client's corroboration. When analogy is experienced by the client, then in a phenomenological sense it is "true."

THE MAN WHO COULD NOT DRIVE HIS CAR

The first time the idea of analogy came to my mind was when I was researching the treatment of Joshua,[4] a client with an obsessive-compulsive personality disorder. My colleague, José van den Hurk, acted as the music therapist (Van den Hurk & Smeijsters, 1991).

Joshua had an intense need for security. He was afraid of the unknown and did not dare to take any risks. He hesitated to take actions, and when he involved himself in some actions, he restricted himself to a fixed pattern of behavior. He did not expose himself to situations that might be unpredictable and could not be

[4]For reasons of privacy, all client names in this chapter have been changed.

forced into a fixed pattern of behavior. For instance, when he planned to make a trip in his car or arranged holidays, he prepared every part of the trip meticulously.

Joshua did not tell us how he felt, which we thought was in line with repressed feelings. Persons who feel insecure become even more insecure when they start talking about their feelings. Because these feelings make them disturbed, they are repressed. Feelings that are repressed are unconscious, and thus one is unable to talk about them. The compulsive behavior helps to repress the feelings.

We concluded from his compulsive behaviors, not from what he told us, that he was an insecure person. Joshua was treated as a person who makes this insecurity manifest by his irresoluteness, his compulsive behaviors, and his lack of expression of feelings.

It became obvious that there were close correspondences between Joshua's behavior in daily life and his behavior during music therapy. During music therapy, he was unable to cope with deviations from play rules. He became angry when Van den Hurk made some variations that were not agreed upon before. Joshua avoided playing on unfamiliar instruments, did not introduce any variations in the well-known pieces he wanted to play, did not spontaneously join Van den Hurk's initiatives, and did not give way to free improvisation.

The way he played with sounds showed identical compulsive behaviors as in daily life. In music therapy, too, there was the need for a predictable environment, which was expressed in a careful preparation of every part of the "sound trip." Thus, during music therapy Joshua showed his "Self in sound."

The goals of music therapy were helping Joshua to cope with unpredictable situations and exploring new musical possibilities. Van den Hurk, in her improvisations with the client, used techniques of "elicitation" and "redirection" (Bruscia, 1987). The first type of technique was used to stimulate the client to react. As a result of meter, rhythm, and melodic line and chord progression, a musical process is felt as an ongoing process in time, and an anticipation of good continuation is evoked. While participating in a musical play, one is stimulated to keep it going. If the music therapist leaves an open space in the ongoing process, then the client is provoked to fill in this space, to give an answer to it. By reacting to the open spaces, filling them up and taking responsibility for them, the client starts experimenting in an analogous "field of play" (see also Kenny, 1989). In the treatment of Joshua, Van den Hurk gradually introduced open spaces more suddenly. This stimulated Joshua to react spontaneously.

With "redirection" techniques, Van den Hurk introduced new musical motifs, intensified the musical play, and destabilized existing patterns. Joshua was transported into musical territories he had never experienced before. After some time, he himself initiated musical redirections.

This example shows that in the musical interaction process, the client experienced how to cope with unpredictability, and to experiment with new behavior. After some time, Joshua reassured by verbal comments that in the musical process he had encountered the insecurity of everyday life, and had been able to conquer it. The musical process made possible an analogous experience and an analogous development.

THE WOMAN WHO STRUGGLED WITH HER MOTHER

A second example is about the case of Amy, a client with symptoms of anorexia nervosa (Smeijsters & Van den Hurk, 1993). At a certain stage in therapy, Amy played alternating between the vibraphone and the temple blocks. As a theme of this play, she had chosen "the relationship with my mother." On the vibraphone, she played a very quick and restless rising and falling line of melodic intervals. On the temple blocks, she played a stiff melodic motif. The musical play on both instruments was characterized by repetition without variation. Also, the alternation between the two instruments did not change.

The melodic line on the vibraphone went up and down, restless but unchanged, as if over and over again Amy was repeating the same vain attempts. Someone who tries to make contact in such a stereotyped way cannot reach somebody else when she is not able to change her form of communication. The other person on the temple blocks cannot be reached by what is happening on the vibraphone, and therefore sticks to a noninviting and resisting attitude.

In her musical role-play, Amy expressed the relationship with her mother in musical schemes. The interesting point here is that in her play on the vibraphone and temple blocks she could sound both persons, the one trying to make contact and the other not reacting to this.

The restless, repetitive advances Amy made to contact her mother, she expressed in music in an analogous way. Her restlessness and repetitive rapprochement were expressed by means of a quick tempo, melodic and rhythmic motifs that did not develop, and a musical form that was an endless repetition without any rests. Amy's unapproachable mother was expressed in a tight, closed, immovable musical form, which consisted of a fixed melodic and rhythmic motif that was repeated like a machine gun, without any variation, without any openness to join.

The music therapy treatment process was aimed to change Amy's behavior. Because Amy played herself as well as her mother, she became able to reflect on her own style of rapprochement. Before she came to music therapy, she projected stubbornness on her mother. By changing roles, she experienced that she herself in her behavior left little room for her mother to join. From Van den Hurk (the music therapist), she learned how she could change her musical behavior in a way that enabled her to make spaces where another person could interject (see Bruscia, 1987, for "making spaces").

What is important in this case is that the evident symbolization of her mother's behavior in the stubborn music on the temple blocks, was based on analogy. An analogy goes one step further than saying just that music represents a person or an event (see Bruscia, 1987). The cognitive identification of music as a representation of something else is one part of the story. The other part of the story is the analogy between the musical parameters and the vitality affects of feeling that makes it possible for us to directly experience our feeling when listening to the music. Thus Amy "sounded" her mother's feelings towards her, i.e., the feelings she projected towards her mother.

Both processes, the psychological and the musical, should be described carefully and linked closely to each other. In the history of music therapy, it seems as if one group of music therapists stresses the psychological processes in the clients (such as projection and symbolization), whereas another group gives more attention to the musical processes. What is needed is connecting the psychological and musical processes and showing that psychological processes sound in musical processes, because the psyche and the music both share the same parameters.

A FIGHT BETWEEN MOTHER AND DAUGHTER

The next example will be taken from the treatment of Helen, a little girl of 7 with behavioral disturbances (Smeijsters & Storm, 1997/1998). Helen was referred to verbal psychotherapy because of enuresis.

From her birth, the relationship with her mother had been disturbed in several ways. The child was born by a Caesarean section, which resulted in giving her to her mother some days later. Helen cried a lot, and her mother could not stand this crying which went on for several weeks. Her mother also was unable to breast-feed her.

There was a second reason why the contact between mother and Helen was disrupted. Mother's relationship with her mother (Helen's grandmother) had been developed wrongly from the very start. Because mother's birth had been preterm, she was handed over to her grandmother after six months. This grandmother never accepted the child emotionally. There was a close parallel between the relationship of Helen and her mother and the relationship between Helen's mother and her mother's grandmother. It had been difficult for Helen's mother, who herself never had been accepted, to feel close to her own child, who was born by a Caesarean section, screamed a lot, and could not be breast-fed.

One hypothesis we generated was that Helen felt that she could not be certain about her mother's empathy toward her. When a second child, Edith, was announced, Helen's enuresis, which had disappeared, started again. After Edith had been born, the relationship between Helen and her mother became characterized by a lack of obedience and quarrel. In the contact with Edith, Helen took over mother's role of parent. By taking over the parental role, she crossed the boundary between generations. As a result, her mother lost her influence little by little and was pushed into the background. Her family seemed to be a recapitulation of her own childhood. While mother reacted with weakness, Helen, who deep inside felt weak too, reacted with strength.

In music therapy, Helen had no eye contact with her mother and did not want to play together with her. Sometimes she grasped her sticks and withheld her mother from playing, or she handed over an instrument to her mother she herself did not like. Many times mother and Helen started to quarrel, and it seemed as if mother each time lost the fight.

In her musical play the mother sounded pitchless and weak; she did not seem to exist. When Hans Storm (the music therapist) asked the mother to play a musical solo, her play could not be distinguished from the tutti play. She was unable to express her personality in music. Helen reacted to her mother's submissive role by belittling her even more. When Edith, now 3 years old, was present, Helen acted as a mother to her.

When playing a musical play called "spaceship," where mother was appointed by Storm to play the role of the captain who, by a crescendo, should take off, Helen played very loud, not accepting her mother's leading role. Many times, Helen rejected or changed the direction of her mother's musical play.

In the behaviors of Helen and her mother, specific (in the music) and nonspecific analogies were seen and heard. Specific analogies occurred when the mother, by playing pitchlessly and softly, illustrated her weak position, and when Helen during musical play, by dynamically interfering with her mother's play, expressed her dominance. Nonspecific analogies, which show analogies not in the music itself, happened when, for example, Helen grasped her mother's sticks and when she instructed Edith how to play. In these cases, the analogy became visible not in the musical behavior itself, but in behavior that preceded or followed the musical play form.

To encounter the problem of hierarchy and conflict between mother and Helen, Storm developed musical play forms that stimulated mother and Helen to make an alliance to reach a common goal or to form a coalition to fight the music therapist. For instance, when they sang a song called "Toddle Men," Storm played the song on his guitar, Helen played on a wooden drum, and her mother, on a split drum. When playing and singing together, they all formed an alliance where the child played the meter and the mother played the rhythm of the song. After some time, mother and Helen even came closer to each other when they played the rhythm together. At that time, they were able musically to do the same thing, without quarreling and fighting.

After this playing together, Storm introduced a musical play where he started with a rhythmic motif that had to be answered by a rhythmic three-tone motive played by mother and Helen synchronously. It was called the "Boom-Boom-Boom" play (first introduced by the Dutch music therapist Theo van der Poel). It looked like a musical exercise, but in essence it was a play to bring mother and Helen together. Because Storm, in his intro, made a lot of variations, this play was very funny, and there was a lot of laughter. Storm tried to confuse mother and Helen, who had to be very attentive to his tricks. They only could succeed and oppose his challenges when they formed a coalition. Mother and Helen looked at and listened carefully to each other, and were able to react synchronously in time. In the musical process, an analog interaction process was unfolding.

THE WOMAN WHO LOCKED HERSELF IN A CAGE

Another example from my own research is the case of Ingrid, a mildly depressed woman with low self-esteem (Smeijsters & Van den Hurk, 1999; Smeijsters, 1999a).

Ingrid was an insecure woman who had found herself a way out by giving herself a mask of strength. But she could find no rest in herself. She had no continuous motorial, emotional, and social identity, and encountered great difficulties in expressing her personal needs.

Since her childhood, she had learned to be very submissive. She herself said that "aggression has been unlearned." Her verbal behavior showed a rationalizing attitude that she had adopted long ago. She presented herself as strong and phlegmatic and repressed her feelings, but sometimes—as if it were a "Fehlleistung"—she suddenly revolted in an outburst, which afterwards made her feel guilty.

Ingrid longed to be able to play the piano. However, when she was invited to do so by Van den Hurk (the music therapist), she answered by saying, "I cannot read notes, I am unable to find a melody, and my hand does not work quite well." In her piano playing, Ingrid expressed her perfectionist attitude. When she was persuaded to play, without being accompanied by Van den Hurk, she restlessly searched for a classical melodic line. Although Ingrid wanted to play a personal melodic line, she did not give herself enough rest to find it. She kept trying but could not find it spontaneously. Because of not finding the right melody right away, she became very disturbed, shook her head, stopped playing, and described her musical play as stupid. Ingrid also made comments such as, "Who am I? In the past I acted like on a stage but lost myself." Not finding a personal melody turned out to be analogous to not finding a personal identity.

In the improvisation, Ingrid did not join when Van den Hurk was playing loud and fast. However, after the musical interplay had been closed silently, Ingrid spontaneously made loud sounds on the instrument. They resembled the abrupt crescendi she made with her voice during verbal communication. She also played on the musical instruments at the same time as she was telling Van den Hurk that she never would allow herself to be "seduced" musically. These spontaneous eruptions showed an unconscious need to express her feelings. There was a conflict between her verbal and nonverbal behaviors, which expressed a conflict in emotional life.

When Ingrid was singing, she was very hesitant and insecure. She herself described it as "laborious." The laborious way she sang illustrated her difficulties with expressing her personal identity. Her voice being blocked meant that her personal identity being blocked. She herself spontaneously connected her musical playing and experiences during music therapy to behaviors and experiences outside music therapy (the excerpts have been taken from Smeijsters, 1999a):

About Her Restless Behavior

Ingrid's statement from Session 8: "I ask myself why I write the way I do. Why is it so restless, why can't it be quiet? Always, I am hewing things down. It resembles my behavior in music. Playing the piano is like my life ..."

About Her Conflict Between Ratio and Feeling

Ingrid's statement from Session 10: "Using my voice costs me a lot of effort. It is oppressive, my voice is so locked. ... There is a lot of energy that is not coming out."

Ingrid's statement from Session 13: "Writing down feelings on paper feels like stepping over a high threshold. I have the same feelings during music therapy. Inside me, something blocks my feelings. ... Especially in music therapy, my feelings are evoked, and then I can feel a block."

Ingrid's statement from Session 18: "I want to sing through something. What is this? Is it aggression, pain? It happens every time when I am in music therapy. I just want to sing a simple melody without feeling anything, and then strong feelings come up."

About the Transfer of the Effect of Music Therapy

Ingrid's statement from Session 21: "There was rest, balance, complete harmony, no tension, no nervousness, no questions, and no negative feelings.

Last week, I tried to stay connected with this feeling. ... Each time when I become insecure, I say to myself: Stay close to your feelings."

Ingrid's statement from Session 22: "I experienced life, going up and down, with highlights and setbacks. In the music playing, I experienced being moved as in life, but without the big discrepancies between hills and valleys. In the subtle passages, I found a part of my inner Self that is deep feeling, tenderness, and love ..."

During treatment, analogous musical processes helped Ingrid to explore feelings and make contact in a less distancing way. When Van den Hurk used "grounding" techniques (see Bruscia, 1987) on the piano, it was possible for Ingrid to find a melody, which expressed personal feelings. Playing and singing a "melody" became more or less identical to finding a personal identity. Ingrid discovered how to play with musical continuation and ease: without sudden breaks, with flowing melodic lines, with rests, and synchronizing her play with Van den Hurk's musical play.

Ingrid was dissatisfied with her behavior when someone else upset her, but she suppressed her feeling. To change this behavior, Van den Hurk instructed Ingrid to react musically when events in music therapy upset her. Thus Van den Hurk created an analogous situation. Intentionally, Van den Hurk disturbed Ingrid's play by "redirection" techniques such as "destabilizing" and "intensifying" (Bruscia). Van den Hurk disrupted the rhythmical flow and played loud and fast clusters several times. Ingrid first became overwhelmed by this, but kept stable and gradually experienced how she herself could use techniques of redirection to influence Van den Hurk's play (changing the instrument, playing as loud as the music therapist, using crescendi and sforzati at other times, using ritardandi).

In this case, there was a strong analogy between Ingrid's rationalistic behaviors and attitude outside music therapy, and the way Ingrid at the start of music therapy tried to play the piano and tried to sing. By changing her playing and singing, she gave space to parts of her identity she had suppressed all her life. This made it possible to find a new feeling of personal identity.

THE MAN WHO PASSED THE 'POINT OF NO RETURN'

The next example has been described by Drieschner, based on his effect study about the use of music therapy in reducing anger of clients in forensic psychiatry (1997, 2000). Drieschner writes:

> "Alan was a man of 30 who had committed several violent crimes. Characteristic for the scenarios that led to his crimes, as well as his

behavior in the client group, was that Alan escalated small conflicts. During these escalating processes, he became more and more emotional (vitality affect crescendo). He lost his contact with reality, distorted his image of other people, overestimated the importance of the conflict, and underestimated the negative consequences of his own behavior. At a certain point, he reached a 'point of no return' followed by an outburst of violence.

In music therapy, there was an analog process—for example, when Alan played the drums and I as a music therapist played the congas. His inclination toward speeding up and playing louder during his musical play was intensified when I played 'antagonistically': more tones, more and unpredictable dynamic variations, crescendi, and so forth. During these activities, he reached a 'point of no return' in the music. He was unable to lower his tempo and dynamics. As in other conflict situations, he lost contact with his partner, and after a short time the only thing he could do was to break off his play.

Together we came to the conclusion that his inclination to crescendi (vitality affect), and in particular passing the 'point of no return,' was a central aspect of his problem. For the treatment of his problem, it was important that Alan in his drumming recognize his experience during his conflict situations.

We worked together by means of a series of exercises of increasing difficulty. First I played rhythmically and congruent with him, when it was his task to accelerate (which he automatically paired with a crescendo). At a certain moment, by a musical sign I took over and decreased tempo and dynamics gradually.

In a second phase, when Alan was able to slow down and make a decrescendo by following me, we exchanged roles. I became the one who accelerated and increased dynamics; he took over control and brought tempo and dynamics down.

Later on—in a third phase—we used the same play forms, but now I didn't play congruent to his drum rhythm, but antagonistically (as described before). In this phase, when I intensified and he should bring intensity down, Alan clearly recognized his experience of the escalating conflicts.

We used all sorts of exercises, in combination with homework exercises and psychoeducation (giving information to the client about his disturbance).

What is important is that the increase of tempo and dynamics—the swelling vitality affect, which in particular but not exclusively was connected to the emotion of anger—became more under Alan's control and less an automatism. He became trained in the retardation and decrescendo, which we called 'to slacken the engine.'"

In this example, we see a strong analogy between the musical parameters tempo and dynamics and those vitality affects described by Stern as accelerating, crescendo, explosive, bursting, and so on (Stern, 1985). As in other examples, it becomes obvious that analogy is not only a theoretical concept but also a phenomenological concept as well, which means that it is trustworthy because the client experiences it as such. For the researcher and music therapist, as stated before, this implies that describing music therapy by means of analogies only makes sense when, by means of "member checking" (see naturalistic inquiry), the client corroborates the analogy.

When Drieschner tells us that Alan "recognized" his experience outside music therapy, it should be clear to us that this recognition was not a cognitive one. During his drumming, Alan experienced the same vitality affect that he experienced outside music therapy. Alan "recognized" the context in which he experienced this vitality affect outside music therapy.

THE MAN WHO LOST HIS FUTURE

This section is biographic, but of relevance for the subject. During the many years I have been researching music therapy, I had never thought that someday I might need music therapy myself. Here I use my personal experiences, and by means of phenomenological reflection shall transform them into psychological language (see Colaizzi, 1978; Giorgi, 1985; Smeijsters, 1997b).

Several years ago, I experienced a heavy burnout. Since I had become a grown-up, I had developed several personal characteristics that can lead to burnout: I worked very hard, and was very idealistic, ambitious, dutiful, and purposeful. I identified and merged with my work, which was a road to existential fulfillment. As a result of this attitude, I worked all the time and gave myself no spare time, which I felt was superfluous, because to work was to live. I believed that I had at my disposal an inexhaustible reservoir of energy, and was able to cope with everything.

But suddenly I was confronted with a situation that had never before happened in my life. I had been appointed as head of studies of several training programs at a time when these training programs, by the national commission of accreditation, were criticized vehemently. Because there was the risk that the training programs would be closed down within several months, in my opinion—and in the opinion of my superiors and the commission—immediate radical actions were needed.

But I made a big mistake. Instead of requesting and increasing everybody's support, I did not await the fulfillment of conditions and started working immediately. I plotted the direction of change and believed that everybody would understand this, commit to it, and join immediately and completely. I worked even harder than I had ever done before. While addicted to work, I became squeezed between the pressure from the outside and the tardy process of change at the inside. I was running too fast, while others didn't want to or were unable to follow at that speed. This trap undermined my energy. It led to a severe exhaustion, combined with a depression. I became so imbalanced that even suicide was near.

When I look back now, I understand that what happened had to do with my environment as well as my personal characteristics. In this part, I want to focus on my recovery, and describe how music changed these personal characteristics.

Music turned out to offer an analogy of feelings of strength that had been underdeveloped in my previous years of life. What made me depressed resulted from an inner weakness, insecurity, vulnerability, and lack of assertiveness that had been hidden under the surface, but in this situation of heavy distress came out. I became the victim of transference, which meant that the submissive role I had taken up during my childhood, which included working hard to try to please others, now was transferred to adult relationships. On the one hand, this leads to exhaustion, because in your own mind there comes no end to pleasing others. On the other hand, when exhaustion is there, it leads to escapism. Then there is the flight where there should be the fight. But how do you change flight into fight?

After the danger of suicide had been countered by medicine and the deepest depression was eased, I decided that I had to change myself. Because an environment is like it is, the best way to stay healthy is to change yourself and your perspective on the environment. To understand the transference, I made use of techniques of psychoanalysis and transactional analysis. To cure my irrational thoughts, I made use of techniques of cognitive therapy. And these therapies played their fair part. But it was music therapy that reconstructed my personality. It astonishes me how music therapy pulled me out of the abyss I had fallen into. Although the burnout was years ago, there is a deep gratitude and affection for the music that helped me, much deeper than my affection for music ever had been.

In my case, the start of the music therapy treatment happened accidentally. Besides my involvement with music therapy, for 25 years or so I had been listening to and playing classical music exclusively. After I fell ill, and became convinced that I needed new experiences, I decided to attend a concert by the Rolling Stones, who—during their "Bridges to Babylon" tour—had a gig in my hometown. I had no special expectations, because in the '60s I had been no great fan of the Rolling Stones.

When the deepest burnout had passed away, I had been playing Bach, Mozart, Scarlatti, and Beethoven on the piano, and it gave me some relief, but I felt I could not get out of it what I needed most. Thus, I went to the concert to do something different. Before I went to the Stones concert, I had no idea whether I could get anything out of it. But the incredible happened.

When, because of tiredness, I left the concert before the end, while walking away from the stage I felt a wave of strength going through my senses and body. The Stones played "Brown Sugar." I listened to the riffs, turned back, looked at the stage, and felt as if my whole life were changing. Although I was tired, since my burnout for the first time I felt real strength. My body felt cool and strong. It was a strength I never had felt before in my life. I went home, decided to remember this particular feeling, and started thinking about how I could use it to cure myself.

From that moment on, I selected musical pieces that came close to the music of the Stones. I looked back at my musical biography and searched for music that maybe could have this same impact and make me less vulnerable, and increase my felt sense of assertiveness. I discovered that there were many pieces I had been disregarding during the past 25 years of my life. They had been there all the time, but they were neglected. I started listening to and playing these pieces on the electric guitar, and made myself emotionally completely open to it. I merged with it and intentionally remembered it before and during events with distress. Especially before critical events, I played this music and "sucked it up." When I drove to work I played the music in my car, and when I went to appointments that could be heavy, I listened to it just before the appointment. Because I was able to remember the feeling this music evoked, I felt different before, during, and after the critical events. I could stand it, and flight had changed into fight.

How was this possible? I gave it much thought. In my teens, I had been listening to rock and blues, but after I had fulfilled my classical music training I was convinced that the music of Bach, Scarlatti, Beethoven, Schubert, Schumann, Debussy, Ravel, and many more represented the highest form of experience. This was not because my teachers had taught me so. All these years, this music gave me what I needed. This music, besides the aesthetic experience it gave me, sounded my vitality affects. This music matched parts of my personality.

But what was it that Keith Richards's rough, strong riffs did to my psyche? The riffs of Keith Richards evoked exactly the vitality affects I needed to overcome my vulnerability. His riffs in "Satisfaction," "Brown Sugar," "Jumping Jack Flash," "Let It Bleed," and "Start Me Up," the songs that impressed me most, are equal to assertiveness. These riffs are analogies of power, energy, firmness, and self-confidence. These riffs are statements that tell us: "This is me, I won't take flight, I am able to encounter."

Unlike classical music, the short melodic motif of the riff is not developed and varied but is repeated, which makes it very strong and sustained. It is not obscured by all kinds of musical developments, but grounded by the bass and drums. As a razor a riff goes directly and immediately into your psyche and your body, gives structure to it, and imprints its vitality affect. It makes all insecurities disappear. As Bamberg (1999, p. 116-117) describes it:

> "The riff of 'Satisfaction' is not 'about' challenge, it is challenge... There is no intellectual distancing... The riff is not about feeling, it is feeling."

I know that the words of the songs and the behavior of the Stones are assertive too, but my process of self-research when listening and playing their music convinced me that the riffs are the essential part. It is not the way the Stones lead their lives that is important, but the vitality affects they are able to sound in the music. Most of us cannot and want not to imitate the lifestyle of the Stones. What we should do is convert the Stones' musical power to psychological strength. And I think that this is the reason that so many youngsters like this and other sorts of music. It keeps you healthy, sounds your vitality affects, sounds your Self, and keeps you from becoming overwhelmed by bad life events.

There is another musician who helped me through, and became more and more important. Eric Clapton's musical expression became my most important alter ego. It was Clapton who said about the blues of Robert Johnson:

> "...it came as something of a shock to me that there could be anything that powerful... At first it was almost too painful... It was too deep for me to be able to deal with... I have never found anything more deeply soulful than Robert Johnson. His music remains the most powerful cry that I think you can find in the human voice, really... it seemed to echo something that I had always felt." (quoted by Newman, 1995, p 34-35).

Shapiro (1993, p. 122) characterizes Clapton's musical play as follows:

> "...there isn't any guitarist around who can wring such emotion from a lump of wood with metal strings. On the top of that he is a blues player, which means passion or nothing at all, playing as good or bad as he feels... (in) 'Have You Ever Loved a Woman?' Eric just spat fire from the guitar, detonating runs and figures that exploded from his fingers."

Clapton's blues improvisations make me scream in sound what I feel. His musical fire, runs, and explosions sound those vitality affects that belong to the essence of my psyche. There are no words to describe what this means. Even words such as freedom, spirituality, intimacy, insight, integration, and being whole (see Amir, 1992, 1993, 1996), are not enough. It is much more deep, complete, existential, about life and death, about who you are, empathy, understanding. From the work of Moreno (1987), I already knew how powerful the blues can be in music therapy. Now I experienced it myself.

Clapton's music tells me exactly who I am. As a lover, this music is able to contain, it helps to express your strongest feelings and at the same time is able to hold them for you. Besides love, this music became the most important thing in my life.

Clapton's blues sounds sorrow and strength at the same time. It is this paradoxical mingling of the depressive mood and the assertiveness of its expression that makes this music so powerful and, for me, healthy. The music, even in its depression, makes me assertive. The long tones, sudden fast runs, the vibrati, string bendings, pull-offs, hammer-ons, rough timbres, and timing of the licks sound power. His music sounds how you can make short, powerful, and well-defined statements. His music is full of emotion, but also "cool" and assertive.

It is the playing from out of the psyche, instantly transferring the felt sense of the vitality affect into sound, which makes Clapton's music authentic and not rationalized or technophile. Clapton is able to transfer basic vitality affects such as being suddenly overwhelmed, increasing vehemence, pushing to a climax, directly into sound. A person who experiences this same vitality affects deep inside immediately recognizes their protonarrative envelopes in the Clapton sounds.

From the moment I started playing his solos on my Gibson Les Paul guitar, my existential anxieties disappeared. When playing these blues improvisations there is flow, there is no time for worrying. You just confidently anticipate the moment where you can break through and make a statement. The flow of sound channelizes your thoughts and feelings in a way that you feel a stream of assertiveness going through your body. There is a feeling of strength that makes you invulnerable.

As said before many times, the client should corroborate the analogy. In this particular case, the researcher has been the client and the music therapist. As a client, I am sure that the music improved my condition of health and changed my personality, because the music sounded those feelings and behaviors that were less well developed.

As a researcher, I conclude by saying that the effect of music therapy is personal and cannot be generalized. Other clients can use other styles of music when they feel that they should sound feelings they want to develop. But in all cases, it proves the effect of music therapy.

THE GIRL WHO WAS NOT THERE

Gindl (2001) describes a music therapy treatment with a 14-year-old girl, Annie, who suffered from anorexia nervosa. She received medication but stayed very depressed and in apathy. One could not be in contact with her because she was "not there."

Annie was only able to play a simple musical exchange with the music therapist on the metallophone, during which she played three tones, the music therapist played three tones, and so on. Annie was unable to change this pattern. Gindl connects this interaction to the very first processes of attunement between a mother and her baby. This process is a very simple process in which nothing much happens. But it is this simplicity that makes it possible to be in rest, to experience security, and to listen to what is yours.

Annie suffered from pains in her stomach after dinner. She allowed the (female) music therapist to lay her hand softly on her stomach. The music therapist then hummed the rhythm of Annie's breathing and adjusted the pressure of her hand, which lay on Annie's stomach, to this rhythm. Annie normally did not look at the music therapist. However, at those moments when the music therapist with her humming and soft pressure on her stomach attuned to her, Annie looked straight into her eyes. At these moments, the music therapist experienced closeness, intimacy, and deep understanding. By the musical attunement, Annie became aware of her own body, apart from the anorectic symptoms.

The attunement was extended by the music therapist's play on the metallophone and piano. The musical attunement was the only way that Annie could be reached when she was depressed, in apathy, and felt lonely. When there was musical attunement, Annie's muscles in her face became relaxed, her breath deepened, and she looked at the music therapist.

When therapy proceeded, at times when Annie was unable to speak and tears were rolling down from her eyes, she participated in a free and atonal improvisation with the music therapist. The music therapist invited her to listen to the music by saying, "Let us listen to what the music tells us."

It became clear that the music was able to sound Annie's feelings, which lay behind her emptiness. By going into the music, Annie was able to express feelings of anger she had never expressed before.

What is impressive in this case is the fact that the client was unable to feel and unable to speak, whereas the music for the first time articulated feelings she could not grasp before. The musical parameters sounded her forms of feeling. The same way she became aware of her body, she also became aware of feelings that had been suppressed. The parameters of depression and apathy were replaced by the parameters of anger. After music had sounded her forms of feelings outside her Self, these feelings could become part of her Self.

This case shows how, by means of analogy in music, the client can find and internalize her true Self. Gindl concludes by saying that when people become resonant for what belongs to their true Self, they will be able to connect their Self to their environment. If a person has experienced who he is, he can go into the world again.

Chapter Ten

RESEARCHING ANALOGIES[1]

INTRODUCTION

In the last decennia, there have been many discussions about research. Some of them I summarized in the book *Multiple Perspectives* (1997b). Since then, of course, the discussions have not stopped (Smeijsters, 2005; Smeijsters & Aasgaard, 2005). In this discussion, I have always advocated an intermediate position, saying that we need all types of quantitative and qualitative research. What is important is that there should be a close match between the goal of research and the research methodology. We need randomized controlled trials (RCT[2]) when we want to know if a treatment group shows an average outcome effect that differs from that of a placebo group. If it turns out that such an effect never shows up in statistical terms, this is not a good omen. This does not imply that there is no effect at all, because there still can be clinical validity independent from research results. Nevertheless, we should try to produce results that prove that music therapy also shows effects when randomized clinical trials are used, even if we feel that this type of research is less relevant for clinical practice.

In my opinion, we should not polarize a controversy between qualitative and quantitative research. Although different, both types of research can be of use and complement each other somehow. So, the choice for the research paradigm depends on which results you are searching for.

The most important criticism of RCTs is that these designs are non-representative because of a lack of co-morbidity, the use of informed consent, and the standardization of treatment (Slade & Priebe, 2002). Wigram et al. (2002), for instance, mention that especially when active music therapy is involved, it is difficult to control and replicate treatment.

Seligman (1995) and Marshall (2002) conclude that the so-called "strong"

---

[1]Parts of this chapter have been prepared in earlier publications.

[2]RCTs are characterized by random assignment, credible placebos, standardized treatment, a fixed number of sessions, operationalized final terms, blind assessment, a lack of comorbidity, follow-ups.

aspects of the randomized clinical trial (the random assignment, the standardized treatment protocol, the fixed duration) give limited insight into the specific process that unfolds within the client and between the client and the therapist. Mean scores and statistical significances, based on standardized measuring instruments, do not give information about the client's individual process. RCTs are neither process-oriented nor person-oriented. RCTs can tell you afterward that there has been an averaged change in a group of clients, which, because of statistical analysis, is not a result of chance. It cannot tell you how and why change took place in the individual.

We may conclude that the weakness of the RCTs is the strength of the single-case designs. The benefits of single-case studies are: the focus on effectiveness in individuals and the process, the inclusion of co-morbidity, the non-artificial setting. What is more, the therapist can be involved as a "reflective practitioner" and the client as a "reflective co-practitioner".

In her article on single-case research, Hilliard (1993) makes a distinction between intrasubject and intersubject research. In *intrasubject* research, there is variation within individual subjects over time, and thus repeated measures over time within the individual. This is different from *intersubject* research, where measures between subjects are used and aggregation across cases takes place.

Turpin (2001) describes single-case experimental designs as a means to proof the effectiveness within the individual. While he focuses on the single-case experimental design and thereby limits the scope of single-case research, I advocate that quantitative and qualitative, experimental and not-experimental, single-case designs all come forward with some type of evidence.

An important related discussion is thus about what we define as "evidence based." Hutschemaekers (2001) mentions that originally the concept *evidence-based medicine,* according to Sackett et al. (1997), was much broader than the actual concept, which has been narrowed down to the effects of RCTs (see also Mace et al., 2001). Originally, the definition included a close connection between theory and practice, between clinical experience and research. Making explicit the tacit knowledge of clinicians, developing best practices by means of consensus-based research, and randomized clinical trials all were part of the process of evidence development. It is obvious that when the research focuses on the cyclic transfer from clinical experience into theory and from theory into clinical experience, a qualitative research methodology such as phenomenology, hermeneutics, grounded theory, naturalistic inquiry, and constructivism is appropriate.

As a conclusion, I put forward that if we want to research the process of change in time and the interaction of client and therapist, we need naturalistic research methodologies in which there is a transfer from clinical experience to theory and vice versa, and that this methodology is evidence based. In this chapter the term "naturalistic" is used as a category of research methods in which the natural therapeutic context is the focus of attention. I will first show that there is a close connection between the competencies of the reflective practitioner, the naturalistic researcher, and the learning student. Then, several naturalistic research principles and techniques will be described. Finally, a qualitative, naturalistic research design for researching analogy will be introduced.

KNOWLEDGE DEVELOPMENT BY TRIANGULATING CLINICAL EXPERIENCE, NATURALISTIC INQUIRY, AND DOUBLE-LOOP LEARNING

Music therapy and the other arts therapies need a continuous development of the body of knowledge (assessment, indications, treatment goals, methods, and effects). In this process of knowledge development, clinicians, researchers, and students take part. Interestingly, there is a strong similarity between the process of knowledge development by clinicians, researchers, and students. Although their interest and scope is different, the basic process of reflection is the same.

Knowledge Development

To be able to develop knowledge, a person should have several learning competencies. Tissen, Andriessen and Lekanne Deprez (1998, 2000) distinguish between cognitive, social, and feedback competencies. *Cognitive* learning includes competencies such as "reflecting," "analyzing," and "creating." *Social* learning includes competencies such as "networking," "teamworking," and "dialoguing." *Feedback* learning includes "sensing," "sourcing," and "questioning" *(see Figure 10.1).*

To IMPROVE THINKING.

- Reflecting: The ability to ponder the lessons that have been learned and developing the art of self-reflection.
- Analyzing: Developing a competency that is based on logic, systems thinking, reasoning, and mental modeling. It is a rational approach to thinking.
- Creating: Requires an emotional approach, as we move outside the constructive box of orthodox thinking. This means allowing our minds to move laterally, creatively.

To BE SOCIALLY COMPETENT.

- Networking: To build up a close circle where we can often find the information we are seeking.

- Teamworking: The ability to collaborate and share knowledge.
- Dialoguing: The ability to rid our minds of any preconceptions and listen to all the arguments with full attention and without trying to interject views or ideas that may arise.

TO LEARN FROM INFORMATION.

- Sensing: Being responsive and open to new information. This means postponing judgment on any matter until full information is available. It means listening with an open mind, observing, and perceiving.
- Sourcing: Knowing where to look for the information you are after. It also deals with how to find particular information.
- Questioning: Turning data into information by making sure that it gives an answer to a specific question. Knowing what question to ask is half of the battle.

Figure 10.1

*Competencies for Knowledge Development**

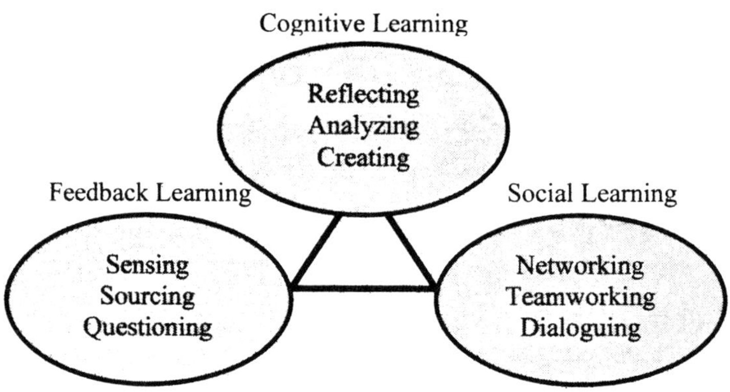

*Source: Tissen et al., 1998

Naturalistic Inquiry

When looking at naturalistic inquiry, you see that several competencies of knowledge development have been translated into inquiry techniques (see Lincoln & Guba, 1985; Ely et al., 1995; Smaling, 1995; Lincoln & Guba, 2000;

Schwandt, 2000) and data process techniques (see Glaser & Strauss, 1967; Glaser, 1992; Strauss & Corbin, 1990/1998; Bruscia, 1995b/c; Smeijsters, 1997b; Charmaz, 2000).

Some of these techniques will be described further here. In the next part, I will give a short description to give you an impression about the similarity between the competencies of knowledge development and the research techniques.

INQUIRY TECHNIQUES IN NATURALISTIC INQUIRY

- Open-mindedness: It is the ability or capacity of the mind to receive impressions, and to undo experience from culturally learned habits.
- Triangulation: The researcher makes use of different personal sources, different data-collecting techniques, and several theoretical models.
- Peer debriefing: Independent experts are invited to check the researcher's data analysis and are allowed to give feedback.
- Member checking: The co-researchers, observers, and clients are invited to comment on the researcher's data analysis and are allowed to give feedback.

DATA PROCESS TECHNIQUES IN NATURALISTIC INQUIRY (SEE BRUSCIA, 1995B/C)

- Analyzing: Connecting data units by asking if one is an attribute of, cause of, type of, stage of, means for, or reason for another (see axial coding in grounded theory).
- Synthesizing: Regrouping data in a new way and developing a higher level of abstraction.
- Interpreting: Uncovering hidden aspects of data, giving meaning to the data, and constructing data within the framework of an existing theory.
- Theorizing: Developing theories that are grounded in the data, but go beyond the data.

Let me give you a few examples of the match between competencies of knowledge development and naturalistic research techniques *(see Figure 10.2).*

Figure 10.2

The Match Between Competencies in Knowledge Development and Naturalistic Inquiry

Competencies in Knowledge Development and Inquiry Techniques in Naturalistic Inquiry	
Sensing	*Open-mindedness*
Sourcing/Networking	*Triangulation*
Teamworking	*Peer debriefing*
Dialoguing	*Member checking*

Competencies in Knowledge Development and Data Process Techniques in Naturalistic Inquiry	
Analyzing	*Analyzing*
Creating	*Synthesizing/ Interpreting/ Theorizing*

Knowledge Development in Education: The Development of Double-Loop Learning

In the Dutch educational system, competencies and competence management have been introduced. Competence is defined as being able to execute professional tasks by integrating knowledge abilities, behavioral abilities, and attitude. Competence management is trained through a personal development plan, which the student during his training course designs for himself. In this personal development plan, he compares the already required competencies with the competencies he has to reach and formulates goals, learning activities, and behavioral products that make sure that he acquires the lacking competencies. By means of the behavioral products, which become parts of his portfolio, he will be able to show when and at which level competencies have been obtained.

Through the process of competence management, the student will become a reflective practitioner (Schön, 1983, 1988). The *reflective practitioner* has at his disposal the "double-loop learning" competencies (Argyris, 1991), by which he knows how to acquire new competencies and is able to "make better things." The continuous development of competencies is required because, as a result of the growth of the body of knowledge, the solutions to the same problems change, and at the same time, the problems a professional has to cope with also change. Double-loop learning is needed because the professional must be able to develop new solutions for old and new problems.

The reflective practitioner is self-regulating and proactive. He has an outreaching attitude and is actively aware of the changing environment. His competence development does not depend on management directives. On a personal level, he is doing what knowledge development aims at on a larger scale: creating knowledge by means of using existing knowledge in a new way, gaining knew knowledge, and creating new combinations.

Knowledge Development: The Triangle of Clinical Experience, Naturalistic Inquiry, and Double-Loop Learning

Making explicit, analyzing, and evaluating tacit knowledge and creating new knowledge are shared aims in practice, research, and education. In practice, it is the "reflective practitioner" who plans, executes, evaluates, and changes his working methods. In research, the reflective practitioner shares his tacit knowledge with his colleagues, is enabled to match his tacit knowledge with theory, and during this process is guided by research methods that are trustworthy. In education, the student develops competencies to plan, execute, evaluate, and innovate his working methods, and to match theory with practice.

What is essential to naturalistic inquiry is also essential in practice. The aim of naturalistic inquiry is to develop knowledge out of experience, to generate theories from experience, and to develop concepts, theories, and guidelines from those who are in the experience. In naturalistic inquiry, a theory is only trustworthy when it is grounded in experience.

From the perspective of the reflective practitioner, a research method only makes sense when it supports the learning process in practice. This means that the research method should stimulate the reflective practitioner to evaluate and refine his working methods, and also to let his working methods become improved by research findings and theory.

In education, students acquire the processes of reasoning that are characteristic of the reflective practitioner and naturalistic researcher, such as member checking, peer debriefing, and triangulation. Self-regulated learning means being able to evaluate existing knowledge, and to create new knowledge by means of interacting with theory and practice.

Figure 10.3 shows the match between a learning organization, self-regulating learning, and naturalistic inquiry. There is a close match between naturalistic inquiry, the learning organization, and self-regulated learning in education. In research, researchers and professionals share and develop knowledge; in a learning organization, reflective practitioners share and develop knowledge; and self-regulated learning brings students to share and develop knowledge. The naturalistic researcher, the reflective practitioner, and the self-regulating student use the same competencies and tools of knowledge creation.

Figure 10.3

The Triangle of Innovative Knowledge Development

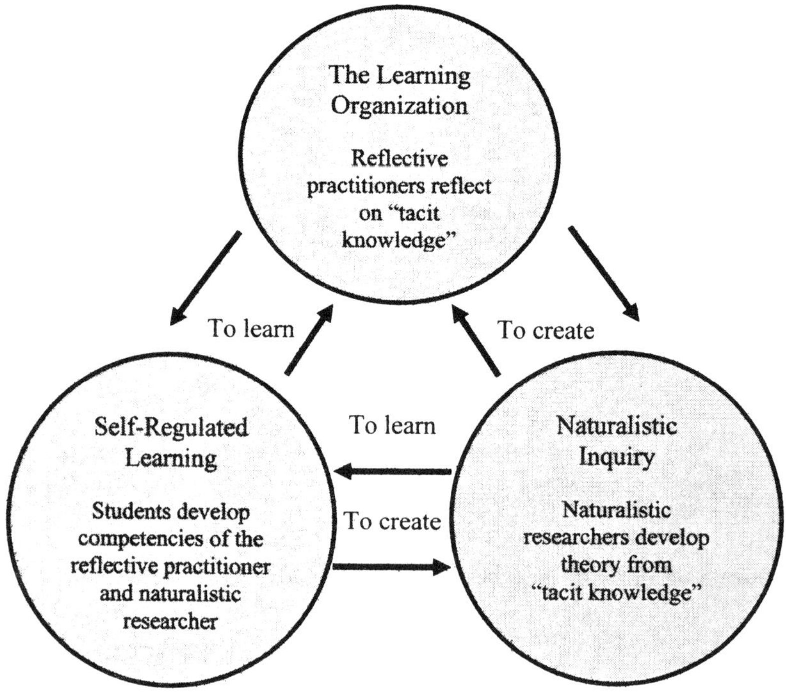

In this chapter, I will focus on naturalistic inquiry into analogies. In the next section, I will start with a short summary of the principles of naturalistic inquiry. Then I will describe a method I use and have used myself with students, with the aim of researching the analogy between musical forms and forms of feeling.

PRINCIPLES OF NATURALISTIC INQUIRY

In this paragraph, I will focus on the qualitative, naturalistic, hypothesis-generating, single-case design[3]. Although the term "naturalistic" in this book refers in a more general way to the qualitative-naturalistic-constructivist paradigm, in this paragraph I would like to describe more precisely the characteristics of the qualitative, naturalistic, hypothesis-generating, single-case design, which differs in several aspects from the quantitative-experimental hypothesis testing group design.

In the qualitative, naturalistic, hypothesis-generating, single-case design, it is the context from which theories are generated. Naturalistic research has as central premise that "general laws," which are the result of an experimental situation in which variables are identified and controlled, can offer us only an artificial representation of what is happening in the real context. Because contexts are specific and complex, if you reduce it to a limited set of causal variables, you do not get insight into the multileveled, mutual shapings, which are characteristic of reality (see Lincoln & Guba, 1985, 2000). In the natural context of therapy, therapists cannot manipulate treatment in such a way that only a limited number of independent and dependent variables occur. For therapists, the most interesting thing about reality is not its artificial reduction to variables, but its natural specificity, complexity, and wholeness in which they have to act.

Replication in space and time is only possible when specificity and complexity are reduced. The idea of sampling and generalization makes sense only when you want to research the reduced reality. If this is not of interest to you, then sampling from a population and generalizing back to the population is not the right thing to do. Experimental research makes possible a cross-analysis of contexts that leads to an abstraction of reality. Naturalistic inquiry focuses on

---

[3]I use the term qualitative, naturalistic, hypothesis-generating, and single-case design because, in a more strict sense, qualitative, naturalistic, hypothesis-generating, and single-case are not the same. "Qualitative" means that the types of data are verbal and not numerical, "naturalistic" means that there is no experimental manipulation, "hypothesis-generating" means that there is no theory from which hypotheses are deduced, and "single-case" means that there is something unique. In the research literature, within the new paradigm research, most of the time, these terms are treated as belonging to each other. And indeed there is a strong rationale to do so. However a naturalistic design can be combined with quantitative data, an experimental design can become combined with verbal data, there can be hypothesis testing in a naturalistic design, and so on (see Smeijsters, in Wheeler, 2005).

the whole of the specific context. Both paradigms result in knowledge, but the kind of knowledge is different.

If you want to focus on the whole of one particular context, as in *grounded theory* (Glaser & Strauss, 1967), you generate hypotheses from the context. As in *phenomenology,* you make use of an "open" research attitude (Giorgi, 1985), and as in *naturalistic inquiry,* you develop your themes and research design while doing the research (Lincoln & Guba, 1985).

"Qualitative" means that the data you use are descriptions and not figures that have been gathered by means of standardized measuring instruments. Because in qualitative research there are no "variables," there can be no measuring instruments for these variables. Λ "thick" description is used, which as completely as possible describes the context.

Qualitative research focuses on meanings and experiences of people in a way that is "open" and not reduced to experiences mapped out beforehand that are operationalized in measuring instruments. This shows the different perspective of the qualitative paradigm. As said before, when reducing reality to variables, it is easy to make cross-analyses in time and space because you focus on those variables of reality that are the same everywhere. Of course, there are variations (that is why the reductions are called variables), but the things you are looking for are the same. Thus, experiences and meanings are forced into a model.

In qualitative research, the "openness" of the research makes it possible to let people tell their own story and thus generate hypotheses. The person, not the measuring instrument, is the tool of research. The researcher, the clients and therapists, and all people who are of interest to the context are invited to tell their story about what is happening. The researcher as a person interacts with other persons, and they exchange and corroborate personal experiences.

In naturalistic inquiry, the criteria of internal validity, external validity, reliability, and objectivity are exchanged with the criteria of credibility, transferability, dependability, and confirmability, which together make sure that there is "trustworthiness." These criteria are met by using techniques such as triangulation, member checking, peer debriefing, pattern matching, controlled subjectivity, repeated observation and replication of the chain of evidence, which will be described below.

TECHNIQUES OF NATURALISTIC INQUIRY[4]

Researching Subjectivity

In naturalistic inquiry, the researcher asks the clients and the therapist to write *self-reports*, and the observers to write *observation reports,* in which they write down their personal feelings, thoughts, reflections, images, intuitions, and so on. This shows that naturalistic researchers focus on the spontaneous, nonstandardized, and divergent experiences of the participants. Because the naturalistic researcher focuses on the individual phenomena as they occur in the naturalistic context, the research includes openness to the experiences of participants.

Experiences are not standardized in measuring experiments. In naturalistic inquiry the person is the measuring instrument and the person's experiences are the data of research. However, subjectivity does *not* mean that this research is a collection of "subjective" interpretations, personal idiosyncrasies, and individual points of view.

Making Transcripts

The self-reports made by the clients and the therapist, and the observation reports made by the observers and researcher, are written down as transcripts that are very close to the original texts of the participants. There are slight omissions but no interpretations. The researcher omits words that evidently are superfluous. All observations, interviews, recordings, and so on are included as transcripts. Because these transcripts are the database of the research, they are as complete as possible.

Restructuring Transcripts Into Categories

The researcher starts his analysis of the transcripts by restructuring the content of the transcripts into categories. Categories are "boxes" in which the researcher puts together sentences and paragraphs that appear to refer to a similar phenomenon (Strauss & Corbin, 1990/1998). For example, sentences about behavior can be put into the behavioral category, and sentences about emotions,

---

[4]This paragraph is adopted and modified from Smeijsters, H. (1997b). *Multiple perspectives. A guide to qualitative research in music therapy*. Gilsum: Barcelona Publishers.

in the emotional category. There can be categories about interaction, thoughts, images, and so on. Amir (1992, 1993, 1996) made boxes of intrapersonal experiences (emotional, physical, spiritual). It is also possible to make a diagnostic category, a category about aims and effects.

In original grounded theory, categories are generated during the research process. It also is possible to make use of pre-established categories (Strauss & Corbin, 1990/1998).

Selecting Sensitizing Concepts Within Categories

Words that have been put into categories can become sensitizing concepts (Glaser & Strauss, 1967; Glaser, 1978). These words characterize important phenomena within the category. As categories, the sensitizing concepts should be tentative. After they have been established, they should be checked by other research techniques (repeated analysis, peer debriefing) to make sure that these concepts reflect the content of the category as closely as possible, and that any bias by the researchers is minimized.

The restructuring of the transcripts into categories and the selection of sensitizing concepts will be done for each transcript (self-report, observation report) individually.

Cross-Analyzing and Developing Psychological Motifs

The previous techniques have been described with examples from psychological categories and sensitizing concepts. This analysis ends when sensitizing concepts within and between categories are compared with each other and put into psychological motifs. A motif is "... a statement of meaning that runs through all or most of the pertinent data" (Ely et al., 1995, p. 150). A psychological motif combines several sensitizing concepts. For instance, the motif depression is a combination of a depressed mood, a lack of initiative, suicidal thoughts, and so forth.

Psychological motifs can be deduced from all sorts of data: verbal and nonverbal behaviors during therapy, client reports made by other therapists, self-reports by clients made at home, observation reports made by family members, and many more.

Developing Musical Motifs

The same procedure that has been described when developing psychological categories, sensitizing concepts, and motifs can be used when describing the client's musical expression. The researcher describes the musical parameters, forms, and processes. Analyzing the client's musical behavior during music therapy will develop musical motifs. Musical motifs will be compared with psychological motifs.

Pattern Matching

Pattern matching can have several meanings. It can refer to the development of motifs (recurring themes in the data), to the structure of core categories and subcategories, and to time patterns of conditions, categories and, consequences (see, for example, Lincoln & Guba, 1985; Strauss & Corbin, 1990/1998; Yin 1998/2003).

In music therapy, I introduced the idea of "pattern" referring to the match of psychological and musical motifs. In this definition, a pattern exists when there is an analogy between the psychological phenomena and musical events. As put forward in this book, the theory of *analogy* states that the musical processes sound the client's psychological process. The client's Self is expressed in the medium. In the next part, we will see how, by means of member checking, peer debriefing, and triangulation, the trustworthiness of the analogy can be enhanced.

Trustworthiness

In naturalistic inquiry criteria of reliability and validity have been replaced by the concept of trustworthiness, which is subdivided in *credibility* (testing whether the researcher's reconstructions are credible to the constructors of the original multiple realities), *dependability* (testing the extent to which all data have been accounted for and all reasonable areas have been explored), *confirmability* (testing whether there is a psychological chain of evidence in reasoning), and *transferability* (accumulating empirical evidence about contextual similarity) (Lincoln & Guba, 1985). In music therapy research, these criteria became prominent in qualitative research designs (see, for instance, Tüpker, 1990; Aldridge, 1996; Wheeler, 1995/2005; and others). These criteria are met by several qualitative, naturalistic research techniques, such as repeated analysis, self-inquiry, writing memos, member checking, peer debriefing, and triangulation, which will be explained below.

What is essential in trustworthiness stems from constructivist theory, saying that people construct a perspective on "reality." The premise is that there is no objective reality "out there" that can be known, but instead ever-changing views of reality in our minds. Constructivism tells us that it is impossible to find "truth," but that it is possible to negotiate about perspectives on reality. This happens in the dialogue between therapist and client and between researcher and subjects.

Trustworthiness means that the researcher's analysis and interpretation should be corroborated by the persons who are the subjects of the research and by persons who are invited to audit the research. By means of critical dialogues, the dependability, credibility, confirmability, and transferability of the researcher's analyses and interpretations can be discussed. As Aldridge puts it, trustworthiness depends upon strong, robust arguments (Aldridge, 1996, pp. 124–125). Each time a researcher makes an interpretational step forward, participants, colleagues, and auditors should be able to follow his direction, and should be convinced that the direction that has been taken can be justified from the data that are available. Yin (1989/2003) calls it the *chain of evidence,* which should be evident. From this, we also can conclude that "evidence" gets a much broader definition. It does not result from randomized controlled trials, but is the result of sound arguments.

Repeated Analysis

When developing categories and motifs, the researcher submits himself to an iterative process in which categories and motifs are redefined when new data come up. The iterative process will be repeated until the moment when there is saturation, which means that all data can be arranged in relevant categories and motifs.

Self-Inquiry

Self-inquiry, or controlled subjectivity, refers to the reflection the researcher undertakes to investigate his possible personal biases that springs from personal motives, views, or theories (see, for instance, Tüpker, 1990; Bruscia in Wheeler, 1995).

Writing Analytical Memos

In analytical memos (Glaser & Strauss, 1967; Ely et al., 1995; Charmaz, 2000), the researcher writes down why and how he made his analyses and interpretations of the data and why and how he used research techniques. Each interpretation and decision he made, each insecurity and difficulty he encountered, should be documented. Then colleagues and auditors can control the flow of thoughts and decisions resulting from them.

Member Checking

When the therapist, clients, and observers are invited to comment on the researcher's data analysis and are allowed to give feedback, this is called member checking: checking the transcript, categories, sensitizing concepts, and motifs of the people we are studying (Lincoln & Guba, 1985; Ely et al, 1995). When this process of feedback between therapist, clients, observers, and the researcher is circular and is repeated many times, it is called circular iterative feedback.

When researching analogies, member checking is very important to establish credibility and dependability. In any case, the clients themselves should experience or corroborate analogies (credibility), and analogies should be the essential products of data selection (dependability)

Peer Debriefing

Peer debriefing (Lincoln & Guba, 1985) or peer checking (Ely et al., 1995) means inquiring into possible biases and testing working hypotheses, by asking independent experts to check the analyses and interpretations. These independent experts are not involved with the treatment or the research. They receive the research report and are asked to challenge the data analysis and interpretation. By doing this, credibility and confirmability are assured.

Peer debriefing also is an important research technique when researching analogies. Independent experts should confirm analogies.

Triangulation

The use of different personal sources with distinct perspectives (the client, the music therapist, the researcher, the observer, the expert), the use of different data collecting techniques (self-reports, observation reports, discussions, interviews), and the exploration of several theoretical models are part of triangulation (Lincoln & Guba, 1985). Triangulation increases credibility and dependability.

Triangulation, as for member checking and peer debriefing, is an important research technique when researching analogies. Analogies should be confirmed by many sources and data collecting techniques and not be diverted by rival explanations. Because the essence of analogy is that the client sounds his psyche in the music, it is very important that the client's musical expression is corroborated by his nonmusical experiences outside music therapy. Very important also is that research shows that there is a need for the construct of analogy, and that phenomena the analogy refers to cannot be easily explained by other theories.

In the next section, I will put together several qualitative, naturalistic techniques in the research of analogies.

NATURALISTIC INQUIRY ON ANALOGIES

Music therapy needs many research projects. The reason that research is limited comes from the fact that most research designs are too big and too expensive, and not very well adjusted to everyday practice. From my own experience, I know that research is possible with limited resources, if you take the right design. To stimulate research in practice, I developed a research design that can be used by practitioners and students. The design is grounded in the qualitative-naturalistic research paradigm as has been described in previous paragraphs (for sources that have been used, see also Lincoln & Guba, 1985; Tesch, 1990; Strauss & Corbin, 1990/1998; Ely et al., 1995; Wheeler, 1995; Langenberg et al., 1996; Smeijsters, 1997b, 2000/2003; Yin, 1989/2003; Denzin & Lincoln, 2000).

In the presentation of the research design, I will use a former student's research project to show that research can be done with limited resources.

Research Question

Are there any analogies between the client's psychological processes and his musical expressions?

Data

All sorts of data can be used:

- Videotapes of musical sessions
- Extensive transcripts of musical sessions
- Extensive case histories
- Transcripts of interviews

If the data are taken from one session, changes within one session can be documented. When there are data from more sessions along the therapeutic process, a qualitative effect research can be carried out.

Research Panel

This research makes use of a panel, made up of practitioners or students or both. All panel members act as co-researchers.

Research Techniques

The essential research techniques are:

- Repeated analysis (analyzing the data over and over again)
- Member checking (discussing the analyses with the clients, the therapists, and the client's social network)
- Peer debriefing (discussing the individual analyses with colleagues)
- Triangulation (using several sources, several data-collecting techniques, and theoretical sources)

The way the data are analyzed will be described below.

Design

STEP ONE, OPTION A: WHEN TRANSCRIPTS MUST BE PRODUCED. Instructions for making transcripts of audiovisual tapes:

- Look at the audiovisual tapes and make individual notes independent from each other.
- Write down everything you experience inside and outside the musical play. This can be:
    - Individual and communicative behaviors you observe (for instance: "The client does react," "The client asks questions," "The client does not show initiatives").
    - Metaphors you experience when listening and looking to the event (for instance: "The interaction is like two cars bumping").
    - Symbols you experience (for instance: "The client is like an unclosed circle"). A symbol is a presentation with connotations that refer to some deeper meaning. A symbol gives expression to what is difficult to express.
    - Stories (for instance: "The therapist is a salesman who again and again offers new articles. The client is an unsatisfied costumer who picks up the product,

experiments a short time, and then puts it aside").

- Total impression (for instance: "Lifeless," "Powerful").
- Feelings you believe the client and therapist are experiencing (for instance: "The therapist feels irritated," "The client is aggressive").
- Feelings you experience yourself (for instance: "I feel depressed," "I feel bored").
- and so on.

These are examples, which means that there are many more possibilities. Observers should write down everything that comes to their mind spontaneously. Essential to this first step is that the observers are open for psychological phenomena. At this point, the psychological phenomena are important, not the music. Observers should postpone focusing on the parameters and forms of music. Thus, even when many psychological phenomena are occurring along with the music, the psychological aspect should be addressed and not the technical aspect of the music. When listening and looking at the audiovisual tape, observers should also observe without any theoretical concepts in their mind, and spontaneously write down what comes to their mind and body.

Whenever possible, the researcher should include self-reports of therapists and clients, because their experiences are the most important bodies of knowledge. If a researcher has at his disposal only audiovisual tapes of the music therapy sessions and no other data from the client's life, the psychological information will be limited. This can be a serious flaw when researching analogies. Therefore, the researcher should collect all sorts of other psychological data about the client. Interviewing the client, the therapist, and the client's social network can be helpful tools. Member checking can be included.

In this type of research, the person is treated as a research instrument, and "subjective" experiences of persons are the research data. From this, you can conclude that in this type of research it is not "objectivity" that is essential, but "subjectivity," what people experience. These experiences are the most important source of knowledge and evidence. The research design is there to analyze these experiences.

At the end of this first step, all personal reports (of observers, clients, therapists and others) are collected and then distributed among the panel members in a way that every panel member receives the transcript of another member and not his own.

STEP ONE, OPTION B: WHEN TRANSCRIPTS OF SESSIONS, SELF-REPORTS, INTERVIEWS OR CASE HISTORIES ARE ALREADY AVAILABLE. Skip Step One and immediately go to Step Two.

STEP TWO. From this step on, each panel member takes the role of co-researcher and starts analyzing the transcript he received. Each panel member makes an individual analysis and is instructed as follows:

a) Read the transcript several times. Then divide the text into little parts that belong to one particular psychological phenomenon.
b) Make categories. Categories are boxes in which parts that refer to the same kinds of psychological phenomena are collected.

An example (*Table 10.1*):

Table 10.1

Categories Deduced From a Transcript Made by an Observer of an Audiovisual Tape

Emotions

- "The client looks depressed"
- "The client shows aggressive verbal outbursts"
- Etc.

Cognitions

- "The client does not attend to what is going on"
- "The client remembers things from the past"
- Etc.

Communication and Interactions

- "There is no eye contact between the client and other persons"
- "The client gesticulates when telling what he has in mind"
- Etc.

The cells contain sentences that have been written down by the observers in their observation reports. When a case study is used, sentences of the writer of the case study are put in the cells.

For instance (*Table 10.2*):

Table 10.2

Categories Deduced From a Case History

Emotions
- "The client reacts in a heavy emotional way"
- Etc.

Cognitions
- "The client does not have any reality orientation"
- Etc.

Communication and Interactions
- "The client disturbs activities of other clients"
- Etc.

Thus, the cells contain sentences of the writer of the case history.

This example is just one of many possible categorizations (emotions, cognitions, communication, and interactions). The choice of categories should be a result of the research data and not be chosen beforehand.

Remember that the musical processes as such are set aside and will be analyzed further on in the research design.

STEP THREE. The research panel discusses all individual categorizations and then decides which categories shall be used in the following research steps. Step Three is to confirm the technique of peer debriefing.

STEP FOUR. After Step Three has finished, each individual panel member adopts the categories that result from Step Three and, by means of repeated analysis, locates the sentences he selected in Step Two in the new categories. Then he starts a content analysis of each category:

- He selects the most important sentences
- He excludes sentences that have no additional meaning
- He codes the most important concepts as sensitizing concepts
- Whenever possible, sensitizing concepts are combined into more general concepts

STEP FIVE. In a further peer debriefing step, all sensitizing concepts within the categories of the individual panel members are compared with each other. Together, the panel members look for psychological motifs. Psychological motifs can be developed within or between categories by means of combining sensitizing concepts (for example, "depression" can be a psychological motif that is a combination of sensitizing concepts from the categories of emotions, cognitions, behaviors, and interactions). Within one category, more than one psychological motif can occur. Psychological motifs (combinations of sensitizing concepts) are coded by means of a word or short sentence.

Table 10.3 gives an example of psychological motifs from a thesis research project by Puhr (1998). In this research, there were observation reports from three observers and self-reports by two clients (father and a 12-year-old daughter) and the music therapist/researcher.

Table 10.3

*Psychological Motifs During Play Two of Session Six**

Motif One: The Daughter Gives No Space

- Observer One: The daughter's play gives no space
- Observer Two: ----
- Observer Three: ----
- Father: ----
- Daughter: ----
- Music Therapist/Researcher: The daughter plays stable without pauses

Motif Two: Helplessness of Father

- Observer One: Father is helpless
- Observer Two: ----
- Observer Three: ----
- Father: This is frustrating
- Daughter: Father loses courage
- Music Therapist/Researcher: Helplessness

Motif Three: The Daughter Does Not Understand

- Observer One: ----
- Observer Two: ----
- Observer Three: ----
- Father: The daughter does not understand what should be done
- Daughter: My start was wrong; I think my father thought: "This should be different
- Music Therapist/Researcher: ----

Motif Four: The Father Waits for Space

- Observer One: ----
- Observer Two: ----
- Observer Three: The father looks at the daughter
- Father: Be aware that I am there, too
- Daughter: ----
- Music Therapist/Researcher: The father is waiting for some space

Motif Five: Bad Perception by the Daughter

- Observer One: ----
- Observer Two: ----
- Observer Three: The daughter does not look at the father
- Father: I wonder if she thinks, "Why does he not play along with me?"
- Daughter: ----
- Music Therapist/Researcher: The daughter continues playing for herself

Motif Six: The Father Takes Responsibility

- Observer One: ----
- Observer Two: ----
- Observer Three: ----
- Father: If I had not taken the leading role, she still would be playing for herself
- Daughter: ----
- Music Therapist/Researcher: I leave the responsibility to the father

Motif Seven: Father Takes the Leading Role

- Observer One: ----
- Observer Two: The father leads
- Observer Three: The father takes over the leading role
- Father: There is an exchange of roles
- Daughter: Father takes over from me
- Music Therapist/ Researcher: Father takes the leading role; roles are exchanged

Motif Eight: Contact Develops

- Observer One: There is a first attempt to cooperate
- Observer Two: After some searching, there is real contact
- Observer Three: There is a turn taking play
- Father: Without verbal communication, find a way out
- Daughter: ----
- Music Therapist/Researcher: The contact becomes more playful and equal

Motif Nine: Giving Space to Each Other

- Observer One: ----
- Observer Two: Giving space to each other
- Observer Three: ----
- Father: ----
- Daughter: ----
- Music Therapist/Researcher: The father leaves much space for her to answer; the musical play was never so differentiated as it is now

Motif Ten: The Father is Less Dominant, Softer

- Observer One: ----
- Observer Two: The father leads, but is not dominant
- Observer Three: There is more contact
- Father: ----
- Daughter: ----
- Music Therapist/Researcher: The father plays softly and tenderly, his play is new

Motif Eleven: The Daughter is Relaxed and Spontaneous

- Observer One: ----
- Observer Two: ----
- Observer Three: ----
- Father: ----
- Daughter: This was fun, this was laughing
- Music Therapist/Researcher: The daughter reacts relaxed and spontaneous

Motif Twelve: Intimacy

- Observer One: There is tender contact
- Observer Two: Much warmth
- Observer Three: ----
- Father: Very quiet
- Daughter: ----
- Music Therapist/Researcher: Intimate, tender, vulnerable

Motif Thirteen: Positive Experience/Happiness

- Observer One: ----
- Observer Two: Funny ensemble
- Observer Three: ----
- Father: Not bad
- Daughter: I learned that I can have fun with my father
- Music Therapist/Researcher: Pleased about contact, happy, touched

Motif Fourteen: Insecurity Toward Tenderness

- Observer One: Tender attempts to make contact, which turn back in undirectedness; being comic instead of tender
- Observer Two: ----
- Observer Three: ----
- Father: ----
- Daughter: Funny reactions to each other
- Music Therapist/Researcher: More challenging play

*Source: Puhr, 1998

In this example, you can notice that by means of listening in a psychological way to the improvisation of the father and the child, the psychological motifs have been developed. What is happening in the musical forms and parameters will be the topic of the next step.

You also can notice a development from the top psychological motif to the bottom of the table.

STEP SIX. All panel members describe individually what is happening in the music. They make use of a technical analysis.

STEP SEVEN. The panel members compare the individual analysis and conclude which musical processes are there. Musical processes are a result of a combination of musical form aspects and parameters of the individual panel members.

In the research project by Puhr, the musical analysis has been made by an independent musician (Binnendijk, one of the teachers of the music therapy training program). Musical analysis, during Play Two of Session Six (Binnendijk in Puhr, 1998):

> "The daughter starts with disconnected bass tones, the father does not start immediately. The daughter repeats a musical motif around several tones and her father starts playing carefully, scanning, as it were, with a few high soft signals. The daughter does not react. After some time, her play changes, and her father joins.
>
> She then listens and waits until her father has finished, and reacts with disconnected tones and a cluster of tones. Then father joins her with a thrill. When they both continue playing, the musical play becomes powerful. Their interaction is made up of short melodic motifs and thrills and lasts for some time.
>
> After some time, they come musically close to each other when the father lowers his pitch and the daughter heightens her pitch. The daughter imitates her father in volume, legato, tempo, and timing.
>
> There is a close ensemble in which both exchange individual tones that together make a melodic structure, which is without a stable tempo, soft, slow, and legato. The father is the one who offers ingredients and takes initiatives; the daughter is the follower. There are several sorts of loudness, but the play is mostly soft. When the daughter takes an initiative and plays strongly, then the father does not react and keeps on playing softly.
>
> What follows is a subtle and vulnerable ensemble in the medium register, within one octave (close to each other). The daughter follows the father's initiatives in dynamics.
>
> The play comes to an end with joined thrills on the same tones (c-d) and ends somehow fragmented."

This fragment shows that in Step Seven, the independent musician-observer describes the pure musical aspects.

STEP EIGHT. In this final step, an answer is sought to the research question, "Are there any analogies between the client's psychological processes and his musical expressions?" When describing analogies between the psychological and musical motifs, one should be very reserved. Meaning should be "constructed" by integrating all data from self-reports, observation reports, and so on. Trustworthiness will be high when the persons whom it concerns (the clients and the therapist) corroborate what has been described and concluded. It is ideal when analogies are discussed in the research panel (including the therapist) and then confirmed by the clients (peer debriefing and member checking).

The panel members should discuss whether the psychological motifs that have been developed in Step Five are connected to musical processes that are the result of Step Seven. As said before several times, the analogies are much more grounded when there are data from other sources and situations, outside music therapy. If analogies can be found, then it can be shown that the client's psychological processes are sounded in the music. Because psychological processes are sounded in the music, it is possible to treat the psychological in the musical.

Table 10.4 shows that in the therapy of the father and the daughter, there were analogies between the psychological change in their relationship and the way their musical interaction changed.

Table 10.4

*Analogies Between Psychological Motifs and Musical Processes During Play Two of Session Six**

Motif One: The Daughter Gives No Space
- Process: The daughter repeats a musical motif around several tones; she does not react to her father's play.

Motif Two: Helplessness of Father
- Process: The father does not start immediately; after some time he starts playing carefully, scanning as it were, with few high, soft signals.

Motif Three: The Daughter Does Not Understand
- Process: The daughter repeats a musical motif around several tones; she does not react to her father's play.

Motif Four: The Father Waits for Space
- Process: The father does not start immediately; after some time he

starts playing carefully, scanning as it were, with few high, soft signals.

Motif Five: Bad Perception by the Daughter

- Process: The daughter repeats a musical motif around several tones; she does not react to her father's play.

Motif Six: The Father Takes Responsibility

- Process: After some time her play changes, and father joins. The father is the one who offers ingredients and takes initiatives; the daughter is the follower.

Motif Seven: Father Takes the Leading Role

- Process: The father is the one who offers ingredients and takes initiatives; the daughter is the follower.

Motif Eight: Contact Develops

- Process: The daughter listens and waits until her father has finished and reacts with disconnected tones and a cluster of tones. Then father joins her with a thrill. When they both continue playing and the musical play becomes powerful. Their interaction is made up of short melodic motifs and thrills and lasts for some time. After some time, they come musically close to each other when the father lowers his pitch and the daughter heightens her pitch. The daughter imitates her father in volume, legato, tempo, and timing.

Motif Nine: Giving Space to Each Other

- Process: There is a close ensemble in which both exchange individual tones that together make a melodic structure, which is without a stable tempo, soft, slow, and legato.

Motif Ten: The Father is Less Dominant, Softer

- Process: There are several sorts of loudness, but the play is mostly soft. When the daughter takes an initiative and plays strongly, then the father does not react and keeps on playing softly.

Motif Eleven: The Daughter is Relaxed and Spontaneous

- Process: The daughter imitates her father in volume, legato, tempo, and timing. The daughter follows the father's initiatives in dynamics.

Motif Twelve: Intimacy

- Process: What follows is a subtle and vulnerable ensemble in the medium register, within one octave (close to each other).

Motif Thirteen: Positive Experience/Happiness

- Process: ----

Motif Fourteen: Insecurity Toward Tenderness

- Process: The play now comes to an end with joined thrills on the same tones (c-d); ends somehow fragmented.

*Source: Puhr, 1998

You can notice that 13 of the 14 psychological motifs correspond somehow with a musical process. What the observers, the father, the daughter, and the therapist/researcher in terms of psychological motifs have experienced can be traced back to musical processes. Put in another way: The musical processes have significant psychological meanings.

Several times, the same musical process refers to different psychological motifs. From this, one must conclude that one musical process can have several psychological meanings. It is also possible to recategorize the psychological motifs and put together all psychological motifs that belong to one musical process *(see Table 10.5).*

Table 10.5

Recategorizing Psychological Motifs Around Musical Processes

Motif One: The Daughter Gives No Space; The Daughter Does Not Understand; Bad Perception by the Daughter

- Process: The daughter repeats a musical motif around several tones; she does not react to her father's play.

Motif Two: Helplessness of Father; The Father Waits for Space

- Process: The father does not start immediately; after some time, he starts playing carefully, scanning, as it were, with few high, soft signals.

Motif Three: The Father Takes Responsibility; Father Takes the Leading Role

- Process: After some time her play changes, and father joins. Father is the one who offers ingredients, takes initiatives; the daughter is the follower.

Motif Four: Contact Develops; Giving Space to Each Other; Intimacy

- Process: The daughter listens and waits until her father has finished, and reacts with disconnected tones and a cluster of tones. Then father joins her with a thrill. When they both continue playing, the musical play becomes powerful. Their interaction is made up of short melodic motifs and thrills and lasts for some time. After some time, they come musically close to each other when the father lowers his pitch and the daughter heightens her pitch. The daughter imitates her father in volume, legato, tempo, and timing. There is a close ensemble in which both exchange individual tones that together make a melodic structure that is without a stable tempo, soft, slow, and legato. What follows is a subtle and vulnerable ensemble in the medium register, within one octave (close to each other).

Motif Five: The Father is Less Dominant, Softer

- Process: There are several sorts of loudness, but the play is mostly soft. When the daughter takes an initiative and plays strongly, then the father does not react and keeps on playing softly.

Motif Six: The Daughter is Relaxed and Spontaneous

- Process: The daughter imitates her father in volume, legato, tempo, and timing. The daughter follows the father's initiatives in dynamics.

Motif Seven: Insecurity Toward Tenderness

- Process: The play now comes to an end with joined thrills on the same tones (c-d); ends somehow fragmented.

This more condensed table shows that musical contact has psychological and therefore therapeutic meaning. The music in music therapy acts as a therapeutic medium because there is a *psychology of the medium* (see Chapter One). One of the important aspects of this psychology is that a musical process has analogous meaning: When people perceive musical forms, they experience intrapersonal and interpersonal forms of feeling.

EPILOGUE

This type of research can be used as a time-series design and assess both changes in psychological motifs and musical motifs when therapy proceeds. When psychological motifs and musical processes change concurrently, then there is therapeutic development, and there is a strong indicator that psychological and musical changes go together. Very important is that the client experience that his psychological change is an analogy of changes that took place in the music. Thus, *member checking* is one of the most important research tools when researching analogies. If the client does not experience an analogy between the music and his psyche, and when psychological changes do not coincide with changes in his musical expression, there can be no analogy. As Stige (1999, p. 77) puts it: "This illuminates the nonfixed relationship between sign (here: music) and meaning, and thus the importance of asking the client for his experience."

Concurrent changes in the client's psyche and his musical expression might be a result of other experiences inside or outside therapy. To make the (analogous) development during music therapy trustworthy, the researcher should also use the comments of as many other sources as possible (psychiatrists, psychologists, psychotherapists, family members, and so on). This peer debriefing enhances the credibility that indeed music therapy contributed to the client's psychological change.

Chapter Eleven

EPILOGUE: A NEVER-ENDING STORY

I want to close this book by discussing several comments that have been put forward during the discussion I referred to in Chapter Three.[5] In this epilogue, I will focus on analogy.

Let me start with some general impressions made by the panel members in Leuven. There were colleagues who agreed with the fundamental hypotheses of analogy, the idea that Stern's developmental theory is essential to music therapy, and the idea that amodality may be a basic principle of music therapy.

There were members who agreed with the idea that music is a transformation of the inner world of the individual and that the client's musical forms sound his personality and current life situation. Concepts such as homology, isomorphism, and analogy were appreciated.

These individual comments give a global impression of how experts in music therapy think about the theory of analogy. This does not imply, however, that the theory's trustworthiness already is confirmed. Developing a theory of music therapy must be flexible, and give space to multiple perspectives. Therefore, it never can be and should be finished. Developing a theory is a never-ending story.

---

[5]The theory of analogy was presented internationally for the first time during the World Congress in Hamburg (1996). At the European Congress in Leuven (1998), together with Carolyn Kenny, I initiated a discussion on this theory. David Aldridge, Dorit Amir, Lars Ole Bonde, Kimmo Lehtonen, Wolfgang Mahns, Mercedes Pavlicevic, Brynjulf Stige, Eckard Weymann, Kenneth Aigen, Diane Austin, and Even Ruud were involved by means of written or verbal comments before or during the Leuven seminar. In the years 1999–2003, I presented the theory of analogy during several congresses, seminars, and workshops in, for instance, Ulm (1999), Aalborg (2002), and Luxemburg (2003). I also invited arts therapists in the Netherlands to discuss it when I was preparing the *Handboek Creatieve Therapie* (2000/2003). All discussions and comments were very fruitful and helped to develop my thoughts. I would like to thank everybody who has been involved at some moment in the process.

ANALOGY

There is an agreement among several authors concerning the fundamental hypothesis of analogy. However, there was the question whether analogy is observable in the musical behavior. As I put it, analogy is based on the same amodal structure that is basic to a form of feeling and a form of perception, and thus is observable in the musical expression of the client. All meaning that is behind the observable can be inferred only by interpretation and using the musical form as a symbol. But, of course, those meanings that are not directly observable are there, too.

Another important comment that came forward was that all suggested correspondences between the musical and psychological world must be tentative, active, and open. And indeed, this belongs to the essence of analogy: Analogy is not a fixed link between forms of feeling and forms of perception, but can be very different for each person, and what is more, should be experienced as such by the individual person. The client, in his relationship with the music therapist, constructs the connection between the musical and psychological dimension. One also could say that analogous meaning is negotiated between the client and the therapist. And even then, if analogy is used flexibly with each client, within one client there is not a one-to-one relationship between the client's musical form and his form of feeling. The client's musical expression implies a complexity of meanings.

There also was the point of view that we do not need a link between the forms of feeling and forms of perception, because music and feeling is the same thing. I hesitate to agree with this, because indeed they are there in the same moment, but perception is different from feeling.

My development of a general theory of music therapy started because the qualitative research I did on music therapists' writings showed that analogy seems to be a core category in the thoughts of music therapists. It is a core category because many music therapists, who do not belong to a single therapeutic school of music therapy, use it. The core category of analogy acts as a metacategory, because it includes other categories and takes a central position between other categories. It also can become applied to different disturbances and handicaps.

On the other hand, I want to put forward that I am not claiming that the core category of analogy can be used in every context, or can include every music therapeutic process. It is my opinion that it signifies one of the important core categories of music therapy.

METAPHORS, SYMBOLS, AND SIGNS

The way I write about metaphors, symbols, and signs has been discussed also. In my opinion, they are different from analogy because their structure is indirect and refers to some meaning that is not sounded in the musical structure. This does not mean, however, that the metaphor, symbol, and the sign are the same. They all are beyond analogy, but different.

An interesting question is the possible difference between active and receptive music therapy. On the one hand, one can say that they both can be analogous, metaphoric, and symbolic. Precomposed music can be analogous because the dynamic musical forms of the precomposed music can be amodal expressions of the client's intrapsychological processes. But on the other hand, in the improvisation the client is freer to express the amodal structures of his forms of feeling in the music. In receptive music therapy, the (aesthetic) structures are already there, and they reflect the composer's ideas of form. Although the aesthetic structures may sound vitality affects in an analogous way, which to some extent can explain why different persons prefer different musical pieces, in precomposed music it is the metaphorical and symbolic richness that counts. This richness comes from the metaphorical and symbolic meaning of form. Take, for instance, an ostinato that supports a melodic line. Then this musical "support" can be understood as a metaphor that can be a bridge to a social context outside the music.

I agree that the metaphorical and symbolic qualities of music, in receptive as well as in active music therapy, only partly can be explained by the concept of analogy. Sometimes the metaphorical and symbolic occur because of analogy; sometimes they do not.

MUSICAL MEANING

An interesting discussion has been raised about my idea that musical meaning is unimportant. What I mean is that in music therapy, the musical structure as it is described in music theory and music aesthetics is not important when it does not include the psychological aspect. When, for instance, one knows that in a piece of music the sonata form is used, this information in itself does not tell you anything about the psychological impact. As said before, then a metaphorical and symbolic interpretation is needed, and needs to be experienced by the client, to show that the sonata form is about two different figures, a development and mingling of these two figures and recapitulation of the two figures in a different relationship. A person can enjoy the pieces of music and the sonata form without any metaphorical or symbolic interpretation. In this sense, I mean that this aesthetic joy is not the primary focus of music therapy.

To be psychologically important, a musical improvisation does not have to meet aesthetic standards. But in receptive music therapy, the aesthetic experience can have an enormous impact on the psyche. When it does, then in my opinion the aesthetic is psychological.

My statement that musical meaning is "unimportant" has been very provocative, and it was meant to be. My intention was to stress that music as such, without the psychological dimension, is not the focus of music therapy. I agree that there are two possible discourses, the musical and the psychological. I want to make a close connection between them both, and to see the musical and psychological as both sides of one coin. But the coin itself should be the focus, and not its sides. If you look only at one side of the coin, you are unable to see the other. Not the purely musical, not the purely psychological discourse, but the combined musical-psychological discourse makes manifest the essence of music therapy.

In my opinion, the theory of analogy also holds for receptive music therapy. However, I would say that what is important is the analogy between the aesthetic form of a particular (classical) piece of music and its psychological dynamics. Only if it is possible to describe the aesthetic form as an amodal expression of the client's vitality affects can it be proved that the aesthetic form can have therapeutic meaning. So, aesthetic form as such is not important. And I would like to repeat my statement that it is not the musical meaning but its psychological analogy that is important. The reason why this book focused on the improvisational music therapy is because its aesthetic form is open. Therefore, there is a better chance that it will be analogous to the client's psyche. I understand the aesthetic, the beautiful that is in each of us, not as a "musical" but as a psychological category. The beauty in each human being differs from the artistic beauty of a work of art. Of course, we might say that every person is an artist, and every expression is an artistic expression, but this obscures the difference between the individual, unconditional, personal expression and the conditional expression of the artist. The person's individual expression is always beautiful. Each mother believes that her baby is the most beautiful in the world. And, of course, this is "true." When Aldridge says that the person is "composing himself," then I think this is an analogy, but not a work of art.

VERBAL LANGUAGE

Each attempt to describe music in words is limited. Perhaps we should not use any words when they cannot in a valid way describe what is going on in the music. The same holds true for processes in the psyche and between persons. Words are of very limited value. If we cannot find the right words, as Wittgenstein (1999, p. 115) told us, maybe we should not try to do so, and keep silent. But we also should not forget that there is a category of words in poetry, fairy tales, and other narrative forms that is not linear, digital, and denotative, but much more acceptable within the perspective of the arts therapies.

My idea of music therapy as a "therapy beyond words" does not mean that there should not be words in music therapy. What I mean is that the music process, be it receptive or active, is different from experiencing through words. I agree that verbal language takes part in music therapy and that in line with Stern's concept of cross-modality there is an exchange of verbal and nonverbal modes in music therapy. But my focus point is the musical aspect of music therapy, and not the verbal. As Weymann wrote, words can be "empty and dead," meaning can be "crystallized ... beyond words," and only afterwards may it be possible to connect the empty words with "touching experiences." This brings us exactly to the point I wanted to raise in this book: How is it possible that meaning becomes established in the music beyond words?

I would like to stress that, although there is a cross-modal analogous exchange between the verbal and the nonverbal, there is a difference between what can be experienced in the music and what can be experienced through words. This is the reason why music therapy is needed.

EXPRESSION AND IMPRESSION

Now, let us for the last time in this book focus on the "directness" of the experience. The musical expression is a *direct* analogous expression of the dynamics of the psyche, independent from being a representation of something else (a tree, the wind, a place, a land). The dynamics of improvisation are the *same* as the dynamics of the psyche. There is no act of *association* needed.

The musical improvisation is analogous to the inner experience, but it also goes beyond this. The musical improvisation goes beyond the inner experience because it not only is an expression but an *impression* as well. It is the *power* of musical improvisation that going into it brings you to new musical spaces and thus new analogous experiences. Because the new musical territory is analogous to a new territory of inner experience, this impression evokes experiences in the person and facilitates personal change.

CLOSING

Let me close this book, which was a journey into music therapy as an analogy of intra and interpersonal experience, by celebrating the power that music can have on our psyche. Music sounds our inner being and our connections to the world. It goes back in our personal history, it gives us hope for a new future, it sounds grief and strengths, it articulates the conscious and unconscious parts of our soul. Music can be your companion through lifetime, when there are no words to define what happened, no words to tell yourself and others how you feel.

REFERENCES

Aigen, K. (1995a). An aesthetic foundation of clinical theory: An underlying basis of creative music therapy. In C.B. Kenny (Ed.), *Listening, playing, creating: Essays on the power of sound* (pp. 233-257). Albany: State University of New York Press.

Aigen, K. (1995b). Interpretational research. In B. Wheeler (Ed.), *Music therapy research: Quantitative and qualitative perspectives* (pp. 329-364). Phoenixville, PA: Barcelona Publishers.

Aigen, K. (1995c). Philosophical inquiry. In B. Wheeler (Ed.), *Music therapy research: Quantitative and qualitative perspectives* (pp. 447-484). Phoenixville, PA: Barcelona Publishers.

Aldridge, D. (1989). A phenomenological comparison of the organization of music and the Self. *The Arts in Psychotherapy*, *16*, 91–97.

Aldridge, D. (1996). *Music therapy research and practice in medicine: From out of silence*. London: Jessica Kingsley Publishers.

Aldridge, D., Brandt G., & Wohler D. (1990). Toward a common language among the creative art therapies. *The Arts in Psychotherapy*, *17*, 189–195.

Alvin, J., & Warwick, A. (1991). *Music therapy for the autistic child*. Oxford: Oxford University Press.

Amir, D. (1992). *Awakening and expanding the Self: Meaningful moments in the music therapy process as experienced and described by music therapists and music therapy clients*. Unpublished doctoral dissertation, New York University.

Amir, D. (1993). Moments of insight in the music therapy experience. *Music Therapy*, *12*(1), 85–100.

Amir, D. (1996). Experiencing music therapy: meaningful moments in the music therapy process. In M. Langenberg, K. Aigen, & J. Frommer (Eds.), *Qualitative music therapy research: Beginning dialogues* (pp. 109-129). Gilsum, NH: Barcelona Publishers.

Andreasen, N.C. (1982). Negative symptoms in schizophrenia: Definition and reliability. *Archives of General Psychiatry*, *39*, 784–788.

Ansdell, G. (1995). *Music for life: Aspects of creative music therapy with adult clients*. London: Jessica Kingsley Publishers.

Anthony, W.A., & Liberman, R.P. (1986). The practice of psychiatric rehabilitation. *Schizophrenia Bulletin*, *12*, 542–559.

Argyris, C. (1991). Teaching smart people how to learn. *Harvard Business Review*, May/June, 99–109.

Argyris, C., & Schön, D.A. (1978). *Organizational learning: A theory of action perspective*. Massachusetts: Addison-Wesley.

Audenhove, C. van (1995). Indicatiestelling in de psychotherapie. *Tijdschrift voor Psychotherapie*, *21*(3), 182–192.

Bamberg, H. (1999). *Rolling Stones. Musik—Mythos--Macht. Geschichte und Geschichten zur dienstältesten Rockband der Welt*. Mainz: Atlantis Schott.

Barker, S.L., Funk, S.C., & Houston, B.K. (1988). Psychological treatment versus nonspecific factors: A meta-analysis of conditions that engender comparable expectations for improvement. *Clinical Psychology Review, 8*, 579–594.

Bärmark, J., & Hallin, M. (1999). Sailing between the Charybdis of theoretical abstractions and the Scylla of unreflected experiences. Some comments upon an essay by Carolyn Kenny. *Nordic Journal of Music Therapy, 8*(2), 137–142.

Benedetti, G. (1991). *Todeslandschaften der Seele: Psychopathologie, Psychodymanik und Psychotherapie der Schizophrenie*. Göttingen: Vandenhoeck und Ruprecht.

Bengtsson, I. (1973). "Verstehen" - Prolegomena zu einem semiotisch-hermeneutischen Ansatz. In P. Faltin & H-P. Reinecke (Hrsg.), *Musik und Verstehen. Aufsätze zur semiotischen Theorie, Ästhetik und Soziologie der musikalischen Rezeption* (pp. 11-36). Köln: Arno Volk Verlag/Hans Gerig.

Berger, D.S. (2002). *Music therapy, sensory integration and the autistic child*. London: Jessica Kingsley Publishers.

Berk, P. Van den (1996). *Questionnaire about criteria for indications*. Presented during the 8th World Congress of Music Therapy, Hamburg.

Bosch, R.J. van den (1994). Schizofrenie en andere psychotische stoornissen. In W. Vandereycken, C.A.L. Hoogduin, & P.M.G. Emmelkamp (Eds.), *Handboek psychopathologie,* deel 1 (pp. 115-163). Houten/Zaventem: Bohn Stafleu Van Loghum.

Boxill, E.H. (1985). *Music therapy for the developmentally disabled*. Austin, TX: Pro-ed.

Brownell, M.D. (2002). Musically adapted social stories to modify behaviors in students with autism: Four case studies. *Journal of Music Therapy, XXXIX*(2), 117-144.

Bruscia, K.E. (1987). *Improvisational models of music therapy*. Springfield, IL: Charles C. Thomas Publisher.

Bruscia, K.E. (1989/1998). *Defining music therapy*. Phoenixville, PA: Barcelona Publishers.

Bruscia, K..E. (1995a). Differences between quantitative and qualitative research paradigms: Implications for music therapy. In B. Wheeler (Ed.), *Music therapy research: Quantitative and qualitative perspectives* (pp. 65-76). Phoenixville, PA: Barcelona Publishers.

Bruscia, K.E. (1995b). The process of doing qualitative research: Part I: Introduction. In B. Wheeler (Ed.), *Music therapy research: Quantitative and qualitative perspectives* (pp. 389-399). Phoenixville, PA: Barcelona Publishers.

Bruscia, K.E. (1995c). The process of doing qualitative research: Part II: Procedural steps. In B. Wheeler (Ed.), *Music therapy research: Quantitative and qualitative perspectives* (pp. 401-427). Phoenixville, PA: Barcelona Publishers.

Bruscia, K.E. (1995d). The process of doing qualitative research: Part III: The human side. In B. Wheeler (Ed.), *Music therapy research: Quantitative and qualitative perspectives* (pp. 429-443). Phoenixville, PA: Barcelona Publishers.

Bruscia, K.E. (1995e). Topics, phenomena, and purposes in qualitative research. In B. Wheeler (Ed.), *Music therapy research: Quantitative and qualitative perspectives* (pp. 313-327). Phoenixville, PA: Barcelona Publishers.

Bryan, A. (1992). Autistic group case study. *Journal of British Music Therapy, 6,* 16–21.

Buchert, H. (2003). *Musiktherapeutische Behandlung bei chronisch schizophrenen Patienten. Durchführung und Auswertung einer Verlaufsstudie zu Wirksamkeit und Wirkungsweise.* Münster: Lit Verlag.

Bunt, L. (1994). *Music therapy. An art beyond words.* London: Routledge.

Charmaz, K. (2000). Grounded theory. Objectivist and constructivist methods. In N.K. Denzin & Y.S. Lincoln (Eds.), *Handbook of qualitative research* (pp. 509-535). London: Sage Publications.

Cimmermans, G. (2000). Werkwijzen in dramatherapie. Lezing gehouden tijdens de landelijke studiedag dramatherapie. Unpublished paper.

Cleven, G. (2001). Van kunst naar kunde. Op weg naar een module schrijven. *Tijdschrift voor Creatieve Therapie, 20*(2), 9–11.

Colaizzi, P.F. (1978). Psychological research as the phenomenologist views it. In R.S. Valle & M. King (Eds.), *Existential phenomenological alternatives for psychology.* New York, NY: Oxford University Press.

Coursey, R.D. (1989). Psychotherapy with persons suffering from schizophrenia: the need for a new agenda. *Schizophrenia Bulletin, 15*(3), 349–359.

De l'Etoile, S.K. (2002). The effectiveness of music therapy in group psychotherapy for adults with mental illness. *The Arts in Psychotherapy, 29*(2), 69-78.

Delfos, M.F. (2000). *Kinderen en gedragsproblemen.* Lisse: Swets & Zeitlinger.

Denzin, N.K., & Lincoln, Y.S. (Eds.). (2000). *Handbook of qualitative research.* London: Sage Publications.

Dissanayake, E. (1996). *Homo aestheticus: Where art comes from and why.* Seattle, WA: University of Washington Press.

Drieschner, K. (1997). *Vermindering van boosheid door muziektherapie: Een gecontroleerd effectonderzoek met forensisch psychiatrische patiënten.* Amsterdam: Universiteit van Amsterdam.

Drieschner, K. (2000). An example of analogy in music therapy. Based on the master thesis: *Vermindering van boosheid door muziektherapie: een gecontroleerd effectonderzoek met forensisch psychiatrische patiënten.* The example has been listed in H. Smeijsters (2000/2003), *Handboek creatieve therapie.* Bussum: Coutinho.

Drieschner, K., & Pioch, A. (2000). Muziektherapie op maat. Methodische keuzes van ervaren muziektherapeuten. *Tijdschrift voor Creatieve Therapie, 19*(3), 9–17.

Ely, M., Anzul, M., Friedman, T., Garner, D., & McGormack Steinmetz, A. (1995). *Doing qualitative research: Circles within circles.* London: The Falmer Press.

Emmelkamp, P.M.G. (1995). Gedragstherapeutische behandeling van angststoornissen. In J.A. den Boer, & H.G.M. Westenberg, *Leerboek angststoornissen. Een neurobiologische benadering.* Utrecht: de Tijdstroom.

Engeland, H. van (1992). Biological aspects: information processing, neuropeptides and behaviour. Paper presented at the 4th Congress on Autism, The Hague.

Forinash, M. (1992). A phenomenological analysis of Nordoff-Robbins approach to music therapy: The lived experience of clinical improvisation. *Music Therapy, 11*, 120–141.

Forinash, M. (1995). Phenomenological research. In B.L. Wheeler (Ed.), *Music therapy research. Quantitative and qualitative perspectives* (pp. 367-387). Phoenixville, PA: Barcelona Publishers.

Forinash, M., & Gonzalez, D. (1989). A phenomenological perspective of music therapy. *Music Therapy, 8*(1), 35–46.

Foster, M. LeCron (1978). The symbolic structure of primordial language. In Washburn, L. Sherwood, & E.R. McCrown (Eds.), *Human evolution: Biosocial perspectives.* Menlo Park: Benjamin/Cummings.

Franco, G. di (1999). Music and autism. Vocal improvisation as containment of stereotypes. In T. Wigram & J. de Backer (Eds.), *Clinical applications of music therapy in developmental disability, paediatrics and neurology* (pp. 93-118). London: Jessica Kingsley Publishers.

Freud, S. (1987). *Die Traumdeutung.* Frankfurt am Main: Gustav Fischer Verlag.

Frohne-Hagemann, I. (1986). Vorwort. In F. Hegi, *Improvisation und Musiktherapie* (pp. 17-18). Paderborn: Junfermann-Verlag.

Garred, R. (2001, November 1). The ontology of music in music therapy. A dialogical view. *Voices. A World Forum for Music Therapy. Main Issues, 1*(3).

Gieles, J.B., Jager, S.W.A. de, & Laarhoven, I.M.H. van (Eds.). (1997). *Van profileren naar samenwerken.* Venray: Vincent van Gogh Instituut.

Gindl, B. (2001). "Anklang" finden. Emotionale Resonanz im musiktherapeutischen Prozess. *Musiktherapeutische Umschau, 22*(1), 7–18.

Giorgi, A. (1985). *Phenomenology and psychological research.* Pittsburgh, PA: Duquesne University Press.

Glaser, B.G. (1978). *Theoretical sensitivity.* Mill Valley, CA: Sociology Press.

Glaser, B.G. (1992). *Basics of grounded theory analysis: Emergency versus forcing.* Mill Valley, CA: Sociology Press.

Glaser, B.G., & Strauss, A.L. (1967). *The discovery of grounded theory.* Chicago, IL: Adline.

Grainger, R. (1999). *Researching the arts therapies. A dramatherapist's perspective.* London: Jessica Kingsley Publishers.

Grainger, R. (2001/2002). Thoughts on the future of drama therapy research. *Dramatherapy, 23*(3), 9–11.

Gregg, G.S. (1991). *Self-representation: Live narrative studies in identity and ideology.* New York, NY: Greenwood Press.

Greimas, A.J., & Courtés, J. (1979). *Sémiotique: Dictionnaire raisonné de la théorie du langage.* Paris: Hachette.

Gunderson, J.G., Frank, A.F., Katz, H.M., Vannicelli, M.L., Frosch, J.P., & Knapp, P.H. (1984). Effects of psychotherapy in schizophrenia II: Comparative outcome of two forms of treatment. *Schizophrenia Bulletin, 10,* 564–598.

Hafkamp, H. (1997). Indikationen der Musiktherapie in der Behandlung von geistig Behinderten. In *Tagungsdokumentationen zum Symposium 'Hast du Töne? Musik und Therapie im Rheinland'* (pp. 22-29). Köln: Landschaftsverband Rheinland.

Hargreaves, D.J. (1988). *The developmental psychology of music.* Cambridge: Cambridge University Press.

Hartogh, T. (2002). Analogiebildung in der Musiktherapie. Eine wissenschaftstheoretische Betrachtung. *Zeitschrift für Musik-, Tanz- und Kunsttherapie, 13*(2), 51–60.

Hattum, M. van, & Hutschemaekers, G. (2000). *Vakwerk. Producttyperingen van vaktherapeuten voor het programma stemmingsstoornissen.* Utrecht: Trimbos Instituut.

Hayashi, N., Tanabe, Y., Nakagawa, S., Noguchi, M., Iwata, C., Kobuchi, Y., Watanabe, M., Okui, M., Takagi, K., Sugita, K., Horiuchi, K., Sasaki, A., & Koike, I. (2002). Effects of group music therapy on inpatients with chronic psychoses: a controlled study. *Psychiatry and Clinical Neurosciences, 56,* 187-193.

Heal, M. (1991). Psychoanalytisch orientierte Musiktherapie bei geistig Behinderten. *Musiktherapeutische Umschau, 12*(2), 110–127.

Hegi, F. (1997). Die heilenden Prozesse in der musiktherapeutischen Improvisation. In L. Müller & H.G. Petzold (Hrsg.), *Musiktherapie in der klinischen Arbeit. Integrative Modelle und Methoden* (pp. 76-90). Stuttgart:

Gustav Fischer Verlag.

Hegi, F. (1998). *Übergänge zwischen Sprache und Musik. Die Wirkungskomponenten der Musiktherapie*. Paderborn: Junfermann Verlag.

Hermans, H. (1993). Music as metaphor for the Self. Review of G.S. Gregg (1991). Self-representation: Life narrative studies in identity and ideology. *Contemporary Psychology*, *38*(2), 177–179.

Hesse, M. (1967). Models and analogy in science. In *The encyclopedia of philosophy, Vol. 4*. New York, NY: MacMillan.

Hilliard, R.B. (1993). Single-case methodology in psychotherapy and outcome research. *Journal of Consulting and Clinical Psychology*, *61*(3), 373–380.

Horkheimer, M., & Adorno, T.W. (1981). *Dialektik der Aufklärung*. Frankfurt am Main: Fischer Taschenbuch Verlag.

Hurk, J. van den & Smeijsters, H. (1991). Musical improvisation in the treatment of a man with obsessive compulsive personality disorder. In K.E. Bruscia (Ed.), *Case studies in music therapy* (pp. 387-402). Phoenixville, PA: Barcelona Publishers.

Hutschemaekers, G. (2001*). Onder professionals. Hulpverleners en cliënten in de geestelijke gezondheidszorg. Inaugurele Rede*. Nijmegen: SUN.

Jensen, B. (1999). Music therapy with psychiatric in-patients: A case study with a young schizophrenic man. In T. Wigram & J. de Backer (Eds.), *Clinical applications of music therapy in psychiatry* (pp. 44-60). London: Jessica Kingsley Publishers.

Jochims, S. (1990). Krankheitsverarbeitung in der Frühphase schwerer neurologischer Erkrankungen. *Psychotherapie, Psychosomatik und medizinische Psychologie*, *40*, 115–122.

Jonghe, F. de, Janssen, R., & Rijnierse, P. (1987). Uitzicht op inzicht I. *Tijdschrift voorPsychotherapie*, *13*, 180–190.

Jonghe, F. de, Janssen, R., & Rijnierse, P. (1988a). Uitzicht op inzicht II. *Tijdschrift voorPsychotherapie*, *14*, 2–15.

Jonghe, F. de, Janssen, R., & Rijnierse, P. (1988b). Uitzicht op inzicht III. *Tijdschrift voorPsychotherapie*, *14*, 91–99.

Jung, C.G. (1985). *Die Archetypen und das kollektive Unbewußte*. Olten: Walter-Verlag.

Kenny, C.B. (1989). *The field of play: A guide for the theory and practice of music therapy*. Atascadero, CA: Ridgeview Publishing Company.

Kenny, C.B. (1996a). Remembering what's between the lines. In M. Langenberg, K. Aigen, & J. Frommer (Eds.), *Qualitative music therapy research. Beginning dialogues* (pp. 191-199). Gilsum, NH: Barcelona Publishers.

Kenny, C.B. (1996b). The dilemma of uniqueness: An essay on consciousness and qualities. *Nordisk Tidsskrift for Musikkterapi*, *5*(2), 87–96.

Kenny, C.B. (1996c). The story of the field of play. In M. Langenberg, K. Aigen, & J. Frommer (Eds.), *Qualitative music therapy research: Beginning dialogues* (pp. 55-78). Gilsum, NH: Barcelona Publishers.

Kenny, C.B. (1997). *Developing concepts for a general theory of music therapy*. Leuven paper.

Kenny, C.B. (1998). Embracing complexity: The creation of a comprehensive research culture in music therapy. *Journal of Music Therapy, 35*(3), 201–217.

Kenny, C.B. (1999). Beyond this point there be dragons: Developing a general theory in music therapy. *Nordic Journal of Music Therapy, 8*(2), 127–136.

Kenny, C.D. (2000). Setting the stage for a general theory in music therapy--Reply to Bärmark & Hallin, *Nordic Journal of Music Therapy, 9*(1), 64–69.

Kenny, C.B. (2002, July 16). Are we really looking for an "Ontology"? Response to Rudy Garred's essay in *Voices. A World Forum for Music Therapy. Moderated Discussion, 1*(3).

Klis, P. Van der (1997). Peptalk in therapeutenland. Van disciplinegebonden euforie naar cliëntgerichte samenwerking. In J.B. Gieles, S.W.A. de Jager, & I.M.H. van Laarhoven (Eds.), *Van profileren naar samenwerken* (pp. 242-248). Venray: Vincent van Gogh Instituut.

Knill, P. (1987). Auf dem Weg zu einer Theorie musikorientierter Psychotherapie. *Musiktherapeutische Umschau, 1*, 3–14.

Kolb, D.A. (1984). *Experiential learning: Experience as the source of learning and development*. Englewood Cliffs, NJ: Prentice-Hall.

Kraijer, D.W. (1991). *Zwakzinnigheid, autisme en aan autisme verwante contactstoornissen*. Amsterdam/Lisse: Swets & Zeitlinger.

Krantz, B. (1997). Indikationsmodel. In *Tagungsdokumentationen zum Symposium 'Hast du Töne? Musik und Therapie im Rheinland'* (pp. 16-17). Köln: Landschaftsverband Rheinland.

Krantz, B., & Poel, T. van der (1997). Indikationen der Musiktherapie in der Behandlung von psychisch Kranken. In *Tagungsdokumentationen zum Symposium 'Hast du Töne? Musik und Therapie im Rheinland'* (pp. 18-21). Köln: Landschaftsverband Rheinland.

Kristeva, J. (1970). *Le texte du roman. Approche sémiologique d'une structure discursive transformationelle*. Den Haag: Mouton.

Kristeva, J. (1994). *Revolution in poetic language*. New York, NY: Columbia University Press.

Kuhl, P., & Meltzoff, A. (1982). The bimodal perception of speech in infancy. *Science, 218*, 1138–1141.

Kühn, M. (1995). *Morphological music therapy and research*. Paper presented at Aalborg University.

Lambert, M.J., & Bergin, A.E. (1994). The effectiveness of psychotherapy. In A.E. Bergin & S.L. Garfield (Eds.), *Handbook of psychotherapy and behaviour change*. New York, NY: Wiley.

Langenberg, M. (1989). Grenzerleben--Probleme und Chancen der Behandlung. *Musiktherapeutische Umschau, 10*, 183–194.

Langenberg, M., Aigen, K., & Frommer, J. (Eds.). (1996). *Qualitative music therapy research: Beginning dialogues*. Gilsum, NH: Barcelona Publishers.

Langenberg, M., Frommer, J., & Langenbach, M. (1996). Fusion and separation: Experiencing opposites in music, music therapy and music therapy research. In M. Langenberg, K. Aigen, & J. Frommer (Eds.), *Qualitative music therapy research: Beginning dialogues* (pp. 131-160). Gilsum, NH: Barcelona Publishers.

Langenberg, M., Frommer, J., & Tress, W. (1992). Qualitative Methodik zur Beschreibung und Interpretation musiktherapeutischer Behandlungswerke. *Musiktherapeutische Umschau, 13*, 258–278.

Langenberg, M., Frommer, J., & Tress, W. (1993). A qualitative research approach to analytical music therapy. *Music Therapy, Volume 12*(1), 59–84.

Langer, S. (1951). *Philosophy in a new key. A study in the symbolism of reason, rite and art*. New York: Mentor Books.

Lecourt, E. (1991). Off-beat music therapy: A psychoanalytic approach to music therapy. In K.E. Bruscia (Ed.), *Case studies in music therapy* (pp. 73-98). Phoenixville, PA: Barcelona Publishers.

Leff, J., & Vaughn, C. (1985). *Expressed emotion in families*. New York: Guilford press.

Lehtonen, K. (1994). Gibt es Entsprechungen zwischen den Strukturen von Musik und denen der Psyche? *Musiktherapeutische Umschau, 15*(1), 9–24.

Lewcowicz, D.J. (1992). The development of temporally based intersensory perception in human infants. In F. Macar et al. (Eds.), *Time, action and cognition* (pp. 33-43). The Netherlands: Kluwer Academic Publishers.

Lewcowicz, D.J., & Turkewitz, G. (1980). Cross-modal equivalence in early infancy: Audio-visual intensity matching. *Developmental Psychology, 16*, 597–607.

Liberman, R.P., DeRisi, W.J., & Mueser, K.T. (1989). *Social skills training for psychiatric patients*. New Yor, NYk: Pergamon Press.

Lincoln, Y.S., & Guba, E.G. (1985). *Naturalistic Inquiry*. Newbury Park, CA: Sage Publications.

Lincoln, Y.S. & Guba, E.G. (2000). Paradigmatic controversies, contradictions, and emerging confluences. In N.K. Denzin & Y.S. Lincoln (Eds.), *Handbook of qualitative research* (pp. 163-188). London: Sage Publications.

Loos, G. K. (1989). Anorexie--eine Frauenkrankheit--eine Zeiterscheinung. *Musiktherapeutische Umschau, 10*, 105–131.

Loos, G. (1986/1994). *Spiel--Räume der Magersucht. Musiktherapie und Körperwahrnehmung mit frühgestörten Patienten*. Stuttgart: Gustav

Fischer Verlag.

Mace, C., Moorey, S., & Roberts, B. (Eds.). (2001). *Evidence in the psychological therapies*. New York, NY: Brunner Routledge.

Mahler, M.S. (1975). *The psychological birth of the human infant*. New York, NY: Basic Books.

Maler, T. (1989). Die intrapsychische Bearbeitung von Konfliktspannungen bei Patientinnen mit Magersucht und Bulimie. *Musiktherapeutische Umschau, 10*, 195–208.

Marshall, M. (2002). Randomized controlled trials--misunderstanding, fraud and spin. In S. Priebe & M. Slade, *Evidence in mental health care* (pp. 59-71). New York, NY: Brunner Routledge.

Maso, I., Atkinson, P.A., Delamont, S., & Verhoeven, J.C. (1995). *Openness in research: The tension between self and other*. Assen: Van Gorcum.

McNiff, S. (1998). *Art-based research*. London: Jessica Kingsley Publishers.

Mechelen, M. van (1993). *Vorm en betekening. Kunstgeschiedenis, semiotiek, semanalyse*. Nijmegen: SUN.

Meltzoff, A.N., & Borton, W. (1979). Intermodal matching by human neonates. *Nature, 282*, 403–404.

Meyer, L.B. (1970). *Emotion and meaning in music*. Chicago, IL: University of Chicago Press.

Miles, M.B., & Huberman, A.M. (1984/1994). *Qualitative data analysis: A sourcebook of new methods*. London: Sage Publications.

Moreno, J.J. (1987). The therapeutic role of the blues singer and considerations for the clinical application of the blues form. *The Arts in Psychotherapy, 14*(4), 333–340.

Mulder, E. (1996). Marguerite Duras en de komst van de muziek in *Détruire dit-elle*. Het verhaal van Bachs laatste fuga. In E. Mulder & H. Ester (Eds.), *De schone waarheid en de steen der dwazen. Transartistieke studies* (pp. 45-57). Baarn: Ambo.

Nattiez, J.J. (1990). *Music and discourse: Towards a semiology of music*. Princeton, NJ: Princeton University Press.

Neugebauer, L., Gustorff, D., Mathiessen, P., & Aldridge, D. (1989). Künstlerin an der eigenen Biographie. Musiktherapie mit Silvia. *Musiktherapeutische Umschau, 10*, 234–242.

Newman, R. (1995). *John Mayall. Blues Breaker*. Chessington: Castle Communications.

Nordoff, P., & Robbins, C. (1977). *Creative music therapy. Individualized treatment for the handicapped child*. New York, NY: The John Day Co.

Nygaard-Pedersen, I. (1999). Music therapy as holding and re-organizing work with schizophrenic and psychotic patients. In T. Wigram & J. de Backer (Eds.), *Clinical applications of music therapy in psychiatry* (pp. 24-43). London: Jessica Kingsley Publishers.

Orlemans, J.W.G. (1994). Gedragstherapie. In C.P.F. van der Staak, A.P. Cassee, & P.E. Boeke (Eds.), *Oriëntatie in de psychotherapie*. Houten/Diegem: Bohn Stafleu Van Loghum.

Pavlicevic, M. (1990). Dynamic interplay in clinical improvisation. *Journal of British Music Therapy*, *4*(2), 5–9.

Pavlicevic, M. (1995). Music and emotion: Aspects of music therapy research. In A. Gilroy & C. Lee (Eds.), *Art and music: therapy and research* (pp. 51-65). London: Routledge.

Pavlicevic, M. (1997). *Music therapy in context: Music, meaning and relationship*. London: Jessica Kingsley Publishers.

Pavlicevic, M. (2000). Improvisation in music therapy: Human communication in sound. *Journal of Music Therapy*, 37(4), 269–285.

Pavlicevic, M., & Trevarthen, C. (1989). A musical assessment of psychiatric states in adults. *Psychopathology*, *22*, 325–334.

Pavlicevic, M., Trevarthen, C., & Duncan, J. (1994). Improvisational music therapy and the rehabilitation of persons suffering from chronic schizophrenia. *Journal of Music Therapy*, *31*(2), 86–104.

Perilli, G.G. (1994). *Subjective tempo in adults with and without psychiatric disorders*. Paper based on a PhD dissertation. Roma: Università Pontificia Salesiana.

Petersen, D. (1998). 'Böse Musik': Analytisch orientierte Musiktherapie mit Kindern. *Musiktherapeutische Umschau, 19,* 176–184.

Pierce, C. (1932). *Elements of logic: Collected papers, III.* Cambridge, MA: Harvard University Press.

Pfeiffer, H., Wunderlich, S., Bender, W., Elz, U., & Horn, B. (1987). Freie Musikimprovisation mit schizophrenen Patienten. Kontrollierte Studie zur Untersuchung der therapeutischen Wirkung. *Rehabilitation*, *26*, 184–192.

Pflederer, M. (1964). The responses of children to musical tasks embodying Piaget's principle of conservation. *Journal of Research in Music Education*, *12*, 251–268.

Pflederer, M. (1967). Conservation laws applied to the development of musical intelligence. *Journal of Research in Music Education*, *15*, 215–223.

Pflederer, M., & L. Sechrest (1968). Conservation-type responses of children to musical stimuli. *Council for Research in Music Education Bulletin*, *13*, 19–36.

Piaget, J. (1970). *De psychologie van de intelligentie*. Amsterdam: Academische Paperbacks.

Polanyi, M. (1967). *The tacit dimension*. London: Routledge Kegan Paul.

Priestley, M. (1994a). Analytical music therapy with children. In M. Priestley, *Essays on analytical music therapy* (pp. 275-284). Phoenixville, PA: Barcelona Publishers.

Priestley, M. (1994b). Case study: Music and the shadow. In M. Priestley, *Essays on analytical music therapy* (pp. 231-239). Phoenixville, PA: Barcelona Publishers.

Puhr, A. (1998). *Nieuwe mogelijkheden in de omgang met elkaar. Een praktijkgericht kwalitatief single-case onderzoek over de ontwikkeling van het muzikale contact in de actieve muziektherapie*. Sittard: Hogeschool Limburg.

Quick reference to the diagnostic criteria from DSM-IV (1994). Washington, DC: American Psychiatric Association.

Rebergen, G. (1992a). Wat te doen met wie? (1). Een verkenning naar zinvolle disciplinaire bijdragen in de activiteitensector. *Activiteitensector, 11*, 1–6.

Rebergen, G. (1992b). Wat te doen met wie? (2). Een verkenning naar zinvolle disciplinaire bijdragen in de activiteitensector. *Activiteitensector, 12*, 9–12.

Rebergen, G. (1993a). Wat te doen met wie? (3). Een verkenning naar zinvolle disciplinaire bijdragen in de activiteitensector. *Activiteitensector, 1*, 11–14.

Rebergen, G. (1993b). Wat te doen met wie? (4). Een verkenning naar zinvolle disciplinaire bijdragen in de activiteitensector. *Activiteitensector, 2*, 15–19.

Rider, M.S. (1977). The relationship between auditory and visual perception on tasks employing Piaget's concept of conservation. *Journal of Music Therapy, 14*, 126–138.

Rider, M.S. (1981). The assessment of cognitive functioning level through musical perception. *Journal of Music Therapy, 18*, 110–119.

Robarts, J.Z. (1995). Towards autonomy and a sense of self: Music therapy and the individuation process in relation to children and adolescents with early onset anorexia nervosa. In D. Dokter (Ed.), *Arts therapies and clients with eating disorders* (pp. 229-246). London: Jessica Kingsley Publishers.

Robarts, J.Z. (1996). Motive and metaphor: Self-processes and music aesthetics in improvisational music therapy with an adolescent girl suffering from anorexia nervosa. Paper presented at the 8th World Congress of Music Therapy, Hamburg.

Robarts, J.Z., & Sloboda, A. (1994). Perspectives on music therapy with people suffering from anorexia nervosa. *Journal of British Music Therapy, 8*(1), 7–14.

Rogers, P.J. (1995). Sexual abuse and eating disorders: A possible connection indicated through music therapy? In D. Dokter (Ed.), *Arts therapies and clients with eating disorders* (pp. 262-278). London: Jessica Kingsley Publishers.

Rolvsjord, R. (1998). Another story about Edward. *Nordic Journal of Music Therapy, 7*(2), 113–120.

Rowan, J., & Reason, P. (1991). *Human inquiry: A sourcebook of new paradigm research.* Chichester: John Wiley & Sons.

Rutter, M., & Schopler, E. (1987). Autism and pervasive developmental disorders: concepts and diagnostic issues. *Journal of Autism and Developmental*

Disorders, *17*(2), 159–186.

Rutten-Saris, M. J. (2002). *The RS-Index: A diagnostic instrument for the assessment of interaction structures in drawings.* Ph.D. dissertation. Hertfordshire: University of Hertfordshire.

Rutten-Saris, M., & Evans, K. (1999). *Emerging interactive art therapy.* Internet Conference on Autism, http://www.autism99.org.

Sackett, D.L., Richardson, S., Rosenberg, W., & Haynes, R.B. (1997). *Evidence-based medicine: How to practice and to teach EBM.* London: Churchill Livingstone.

Salber, W. (1965). *Morphologie des seelischen Geschehens.* Ratingen.

Schalkwijk, F. (1994). *Music and people with developmental disabilities.* London: Jessica Kingsley Publishers.

Schön, D.A. (1983). *The reflective practitioner.* New York, NY: Basic Books.

Schön, D.A. (1988). *Educating the reflective practitioner.* San Francisco, CA: Jossey Bass Publishers.

Schulz, M. (1987). Stereotypic movements and music therapy. *Journal of British Music Therapy*, 11–16.

Schumacher, K. (1994). *Musiktherapie mit autistischen Kindern.* Stuttgart: Gustav Fischer Verlag.

Schumache, K. (1999). *Musiktherapie und Säuglingsforschung. Zusammenspiel. Einschätzung der Beziehungsqualität am Beispiel des instrumentalen Ausdrucks eines autistischen Kindes.* Frankfurt am Main: Peter Lang.

Schwandt, T.A. (2000). Three epistemological stances for qualitative inquiry. In N.K. Denzin & Y.S. Lincoln (Eds.), *Handbook of qualitative research* (pp. 189-213). London: Sage Publications.

Seifert, T., & Loos, G.K. (1989). Möglichkeiten stationärer Psychotherapie der Anorexie und Bulimie. *Musiktherapeutische Umschau*, *10*, 209–218.

Seligman, M.E.P. (1995). The effectiveness of psychotherapy: The consumer reports study. *American Psychologist*, *50*(12), 965–974.

Serafine, M.L. (1980). Piagetian research in music. *Council for Research in Music Education Bulletin*, *62*, 1–21.

Shapiro, H. (1993). *Eric Clapton: Lost in the blues.* New York, NY: Da Capo Press.

Silverman, M.J. (2003). Contingency songwriting to reduce combativeness and non-coorperation in a client with schizophrenia: a case study. *The Arts in Psychotherapy, 30* (1), 25-33.

Slade, M., & Priebe, S. (2002). Conceptual limitations of randomized controlled trials. In S. Priebe & M. Slade (Eds.), *Evidence in mental health* (pp. 101-108). Hove and New York, NY: Brunner-Routledge.

Sloboda, A. (1993). Individual therapy with a man who has an eating disorder. In M. Heal & T. Wigram (Eds.), *Music therapy in Health and Education* (pp. 103-111). London: Jessica Kingsley Publishers.

Sloboda, A. (1995). Individual music therapy with anorexic and bulimic patients. In D. Dokter (Ed.), *Arts therapies and clients with eating disorders* (pp. 247-261). London: Jessica Kingsley Publishers.

Sloboda, J.A. (1987). *The musical mind: The cognitive psychology of music.* Oxford: Oxford University Press.

Smaling, A. (1995). Open-mindedness, open-heartedness and dialogical openness: The dialectics of openings and closures. In I. Maso, P.A. Atkinson, S. Delamont, & J.C. Verhoeven (Eds.), *Openness in research* (pp. 21-32). Assen: Van Gorcum.

Smeijsters, H. (1987). *Muziek en psyche: Thema's met variaties uit de muziekpsychologie*. Assen/Maastricht: Van Gorcum.

Smeijsters, H. (1991). *Muziektherapie als psychotherapie.* Assen/Maastricht: Van Gorcum.

Smeijsters, H. (1993). Music therapy and psychotherapy. *The Arts in Psychotherapy, 20*, 223–229.

Smeijsters, H. (1994). *Musiktherapie als Psychotherapie: Grundlagen—Ansätze--Methoden.* Stuttgart: Gustav Fischer Verlag.

Smeijsters, H. (1995). *Handboek muziektherapie: Theoretische en methodische grondslagen voor de behandeling van specifieke stoornissen en handicaps.* Heerlen: Melos.

Smeijsters, H. (1996a). Analogy as a core category of music therapy. Paper presented at the 8th World Congress of Music Therapy, Hamburg.

Smeijsters, H. (1996b). Entweder--oder? Überlegungen zur quantitativen und qualitativen forschung in der musiktherapie. *Musiktherapeutische Umschau, 1*, 23–38.

Smeijsters, H. (1996c). Musiktherapeutische methoden der gegenwart. In H-H Decker-Voigt, P. Knill, & E. Weymann (Hrsg.), *Lexikon Musiktherapie.* Gottingen: Hogrefe.

Smeijsters, H. (1996d). *Neurologische en fysiologische aspecten van muziektherapie*. Heerlen: Melos.

Smeijsters, H. (1996e). Qualitative single-case research in practice: A necessary, reliable and valid alternative for music therapy research. In M. Langenberg, K. Aigen, & J. Frommer (Eds.), *Qualitative music therapy research: Beginning dialogues* (pp. 35-53). Gilsum, NH: Barcelona Publishers.

Smeijsters, H. (1997a). Die therapeutische Wirkung der Musik--Ergebnisse der Forschung. In L. Müller & H.G. Petzold (Hrsg.), *Musiktherapie in der klinischen Arbeit: Integrative Modelle und Methoden* (pp. 23-40). Stuttgart: Gustav Fischer Verlag.

Smeijsters, H. (1997b). *Multiple perspectives: A guide to qualitative research in music therapy.* Gilsum, NH: Barcelona Publishers.

Smeijsters, H. (1997c). Musiktherapie bei Alzheimerpatienten: Eine Meta-Analyse von Forschungsergebnissen. *Musiktherapeutische Umschau, 18*(4), 268–283.

Smeijsters, H. (1998). *Developing concepts for a general theory of music therapy.* In D. Aldridge (Ed.), Music Therapy Info, Vol. II, CD-ROM. Witten-Herdecke.

Smeijsters, H. (1999a). Feelings of doubt, hope and faith. In J. Hibben (Ed.), *Inside music therapy: Client experiences* (pp. 277-294). Gilsum, NH: Barcelona Publishers.

Smeijsters, H. (1999b). *Grundlagen der Musiktherapie. Theorie und Praxis zur Behandlung von spezifischen psychischen Störungen und Behinderungen.* Göttingen: Hogrefe.

Smeijsters, H. (1999c). The unity of music and psyche: Analogy. In Studiengruppe Musiktherapie Ulm (Hrsg.), *Vortragssammlung. 11 Ulmer Workshop für musiktherapeutische Grundlagen forschung 12/13 Februar 1999,* Universität Ulm. Abteilung Psychotherapie und Psychosomatische Medizin.

Smeijsters, H. (2000/2003). *Handboek creatieve therapie.* Bussum: Coutinho.

Smeijsters, H. (2001a). Die musiktherapeutische Behandlung der Autoaggression bei geistig Behinderten mit Autismus. *Musiktherapeutische Umschau, 22*(3), 204–223.

Smeijsters, H. (2001b). Een masterplan richting wetenschap. *Tijdschrift voor Creatieve Therapie, 20*(3), 4–11.

Smeijsters, H. (2002). De (toegevoegde) waarde van creatieve therapie. *Tijdschrift voor Creatieve Therapie, 21*(4), 9–16.

Smeijsters, H. (2003a). Analogie als Kernkonzept der Musiktherapie. Eine psychologische und empirische Betrachtung. *Zeitschrift für Musik-, Tanz- und Kunsttherapie, 14*(1), 9–18.

Smeijsters, H. (2003b). Forms of feeling and forms of perception. The fundamentals of analogy in music therapy. *Nordic Journal of Music Therapy: Theory building in music therapy--An international archive, 12*(1), 71–85.

Smeijsters, H. (2005). Quantitative single-case designs. In Wheeler, B.L. (Ed.), *Music therapy research: Quantitative and qualitative perspectives.* Gilsum, NH: Barcelona Publishers.

Smeijsters, H. & Aasgaard, T. (2005). Qualitative case study research. In Wheeler, B.L. (Ed.), *Music therapy research: Quantitative and qualitative perspectives.* Gilsum, NH: Barcelona Publishers.

Smeijsters, H., & Berk, P. van den (1995). Music therapy with a client suffering from musicogenic epilepsy. A naturalistic qualitative single-case research. *The Arts in Psychotherapy, 22*(3), 249–263.

Smeijsters, H., & Berk, P. van den (1999). Musiktherapie für Klienten mit musikogener Epilepsie: Eine naturalistische qualitative Einzelfallstudie. In D. Aldridge (Hrsg.), *Beiträge zur Musiktherapie in der Medizin* (pp. 52-69). Bern: Verlag Hans Huber.

Smeijsters, H. & Cleven, G. (2004). *Vaktherapieën in de forensische psychiatrie*. Sittard/Eindhoven/Utrecht: KenVaK/GGzE/EFP.

Smeijsters, H., & Hurk, J. van den (1993). Research in practice in the music therapeutic treatment of a client with symptoms of anorexia nervosa. In M. Heal & T. Wigram (Eds.), *Music therapy in health and education* (pp. 235-263). London: Jessica Kingsley Publishers.

Smeijsters, H., & Hurk, J. van den (1994). Praxisorientierte Forschung in der Musiktherapie. *Musiktherapeutische Umschau. 15*(1), 25–42.

Smeijsters, H., & Hurk, J. van den (1999). Music therapy helping to work through grief and finding a personal identity: Qualitative single case research. *Journal of Music Therapy, 16*(3), 222–252.

Smeijsters, H., & Storm, H. (1997). Die ersten Schritte zu einer Freundschaft mit der eigenen Mutter: Techniken der qualitativen Forschung, illustriert anhand von Beispielen aus der Kurzzeitbehandlung eines verhaltengestörten Mädchens. In H-V. Bolay, R. Boller, D. Czogalik, & H. Kächele (Hrsg.), *Wissenschaftliche Annäherungen an ein weites Feld. 2. Forschungsforum. Heidelberger Schriften zur Musiktherapie Band 1* (pp. 86-96). Stuttgart: Gustav Fischer Verlag.

Smeijsters, H., & Storm, H. (1998). Becoming friends with your mother: Techniques of qualitative research illustrated with the short-term treatment of a girl with enuresis. *Music therapy, 14*(1), 61–83.

Smith, M.L., Glass, G.V., & Miller, T.I. (1980). *The benefits of psychotherapy.* Baltimore: John Hopkins University Press.

Steinberg, R. (1987). Musikpsychopathologie: Musikalischer ausdruck und psychische krankheit. In K.E. Behne, G. Kleinen, & H. de la Motte-Haber (Hrsg.), *Musikpsychologie. Jahrbuch der Deutschen Gesellschaft für Musikpsychologie. Band 4* (pp. 29-48). Wilhelmshaven: Heinrichshofen.

Steinberg, R., & Raith, L. (1985). Music psychopathology I: Musical tempo and psychiatric disease. *Psychopathology, 18*(5–6), 254–264.

Steinberg, R., Krause, A., Lerch, R., & Raith, L. (1987). Das musikalische tempo und psychische krankheit. In R. Spintge & R. Droh (Eds.), *Musik in der Medizin [Music in Medicine]* (pp. 289-301). Berlin: Springer Verlag.

Steiner, G. (1968). *Verval van het woord.* Amsterdam: Polak & Van Gennep.

Steiner, G. (1990). *Het verbroken contract.* Amsterdam: Bert Bakker.

Stern, D.N. (1985). *The interpersonal world of the infant: A view from psychoanalysis and developmental psychology.* New York, NY: Basic Books.

Stern, D.N. (1994). *Mutter und Kind: Die erste Beziehung.* Stuttgart: Klett-

Cotta.

Stern, D.N. (1995). *The motherhood constellation: A unified view of parent-infant therapy*. New York, NY: Basic Books.

Stern, D.N., Sander, L.W., Nahum, J.P., Harrison, A.M., Lyons-Ruth, K., Morgan, A.C., Bruschweiler-Stern, N., & Tronick, E.Z. (1998). Non-interpretive mechanisms in psychoanalytic therapy: The 'something more' than interpretation. *International Journal of Psycho-Analysis, 79*, 903–921.

Stige, B. (1999). The meaning of music: From the client's perspective. In T. Wigram & J. de Backer (Eds.), *Clinical applications of music therapy in psychiatry* (pp. 61-83). London: Jessica Kingsley Publishers.

Strauss, A.L., & Corbin, J. (1990/1998). *Basics of qualitative research. Techniques and procedures for developing grounded theory*. London: Sage Publications.

Strobel, W. (1990). Von der musiktherapie zur musikpsychotherapie: Kann aus der musiktherapie eine anerkannte form der psychotherapie werden? *Musiktherapeutische Umschau, 11*(4), 313–338.

Summer, L. (1996). *Music: The new age elixir*. Amherst, NY: Prometheus Books.

Tang, W., Yao, X., & Zheng, Z. (1994). The rehabilitative effect of music therapy for residual schizophrenia. *British Journal of Psychiatry, 165* (supplement 24), 38–44.

Tesch, R. (1990). *Qualitative research: Analysis types and software tools*. New York, NY: Falmer.

Thoomes-Vreugdenhil, A. (2000a). Relationeel gestoord en hechtingsgestoord. *Tijdschrift voor de Vereniging voor Kinder- en Jeugdpsychotherapie, 3*, 6–20.

Thoomes-Vreugdenhil, A. (2000b). Differentiatietherapie en fasetherapie. Behandelwijzen voor verwaarlozingsproblematiek. *Tijdschrift voor de Vereniging voor Kinder- en Jeugdpsychotherapie, 3*, 20–37.

Thürlemann, F. (1982). *Paul Klee: Analyse sémiotique de trois peintures*. Lausanne: L' Age d'Homme.

Timmermann, T., Scheytt-Hölzer, N., Bauer, S., & Kächele, H. (1991). Musiktherapeutische Einzelfall-Prozessforschung: Entwicklung und Aufbau eines Forschungsfeldes. *Psychotherapie, Psychosomatik und medizinische Psychologie, 41*, 385–391.

Tissen, R., Andriessen, D., & Lekanne Deprez, F. (1998). *Value-based knowledge management: Creating the 21st century company*. Amsterdam: Addison Wesley Longman.

Tissen, R., Andriessen, D., & Lekanne Deprez, F. (2000). *The knowledge dividend. Creating high performance companies through value based knowledge management*. London: Financial Times/Prentice Hall.

Tüpker, R. (1988/1996). *Ich singe was ich nicht sagen kann*. Regensburg:

Gustav Bosse Verlag.
Tüpker, R. (1990). Auf der Suche nach angemessenen Formen wissenschaftlichen Vorgehens in kunsttherapeutischer Forschung. In P. Petersen (Hrsg.), *Ansätze kunsttherapeutischer Forschung* (pp. 71-86). Berlin: Springer-Verlag.
Tüpker, D. (1996). Nichts ist ohne Grund: Musiktherapie bei funktionellen Störungen. In R. Tüpker (Hrsg.), *Konzeptentwicklung musiktherapeutischer Praxis und Forschung* (pp. 8-37). Münster: Lit Verlag.
Turpin, G. (2001). Single case methodology and psychotherapy evaluation: From research to practice. In C. Mace, S. Moorey, & B. Roberts (Eds.), *Evidence in the psychological therapies* (pp. 91-113). New York, NY: Brunner Routledge.
Verhey, F. (1997). Samenwerking en afstemming tussen vaktherapie en psychotherapie. *Tijdschrift voor Creatieve Therapie*, *3*, 3–8.
Verhey, F., & Van Loon, H. (1993). Aan autisme verwante contactstoornissen: een ontwikkelingspsychopathologische benadering als model voor hulp op maat. *Tijdschrift voor Psychiatrie*, *35*(9), 577–589.
Wampold, B.E. (1997). Methodological problems in identifying efficacious psychotherapies. *Psychotherapy Research*, *7*(1), 21–43.
Wasylenki, D.A. (1992). Psychotherapy of schizophrenia revisited. *Hospital and Community Psychiatry*, *43*(2), 123–127.
Weber, C. (1991). Musiktherapie als therapeutische Möglichkeit beim autistischen Syndrom. *Zeitschrift für Musik-, Tanz- und Kunsttherapie*, *2*, 66–74.
Weber, C. (1996). Autismusforschung in der Musik und Tanztherapie: Demonstration eines Untersuchungs und Auswertungsverfahrens. *Zeitschrift für Musik-, Tanz-, und Kunsttherapie*, *7*, 1–10.
Weymann, E. (1990). Kunstanaloges Vorgehen in der Musiktherapie. In I. Frohne-Hagemann (Hrsg.), *Musik und Gestalt* (pp. 49-68). Paderborn: Junfermann-Verlag.
Wheeler, B.L. (1983). A psychotherapeutic classification of music therapy practices: A continuum of procedures. *Music Therapy Perspectives*, *1*, 8–16.
Wheeler, B.L. (1987). Levels of therapy: The classification of music therapy goals. *Music Therapy*, 6(2), 39–49.
Wheeler, B.L. (Ed.). (1995). *Music therapy research: Quantitative and qualitative perspectives*. Phoenixville, PA: Barcelona Publishers.
Wheeler, B.L. (Ed.). (2005). *Music therapy research: Quantitative and qualitative perspectives*. Gilsum, NH: Barcelona Publishers.
Wigram, T., & De Backer, J. (Eds.). (1999). *Clinical applications of music therapy in psychiatry*. London: Jessica Kingsley Publishers.
Wigram, T., & De Backer, J. (Eds.). (1999). *Clinical applications of music therapy in developmental disability, pediatrics and neurology*. London: Jessica Kingsley Publishers.

Wigram, T., Nygaard Pedersen, I., & Bonde, L.O. (2002). *A comprehensive guide to music therapy: Theory, clinical practice, research and training.* London: Jessica Kingsley Publishers.

Wilber, K. (1987). *Das Spektrum des Bewußtseins*. Bern: Scherz Verlag.

Wittgenstein, L. (1999). *Tractatus logico-philosophicus*. Frankfurt am Main: Suhrkamp Verlag.

Wolberg, I.R. (1977). *The technique of psychotherapy*. New York, NY: Grune & Stratton.

Yang, W.Y., Li, Z., Weng, Y.Z., Zhang, H.Y. & Ma, B. (1998). Psychosocial rehabilitation effects of music therapy in chronic schizophrena. *Journal of Psychiatry, 8*, 38-40.

Yin, R.K. (1989/2003). *Case study research: Design and methods*. London: Sage Publications.

INDEX

AUTHORS

Adorno, 34
Aigen, 31, 60, 92, 94, 181
Aldridge, 7, 11, 31, 59, 74, 97, 165, 166, 181, 184
Alvin, 7, 25
Amir, 31, 50, 148, 164, 181
Andreasen, 22
Andriessen, 155
Ansdell, 11, 101
Anthony, 22
Argyris, 13, 158
Austin, 31, 181

Bach, 146
Bamberg, 148
Bärmark, 31
Bauer, 60
Beethoven, 44, 91, 146
Behne, 4
Benedetti, 23
Bender, 22
Benenzon, 12
Bengtsson, 102
Berger, 25
Binnendijk, 176
Boethius, 90
Bolay, 11
Boller, 11
Bonde, 31, 95, 96, 181
Borton, 67
Boxill, 7
Brandt, 59
Broch, 44
Brownell, 25
Bruhn, 6
Bruscia, 6, 7, 9, 17, 18, 59, 78, 79, 102, 103, 107, 119, 121, 122, 137, 139, 143, 157, 166
Bryan, 25
Buchert, 23
Bunt, 74

Clapton, 148-149
Clynes, 4
Colaizzi, 145
Corbin, 57, 61, 157, 163, 165, 168
Coursey, 22
Courtés, 81
Czogalik, 11

Debussy, 147
Decker-Voigt, 6
De Jager, 17
De l'Etoile, 23
Delfos, 26
DeRisi, 22
Deutsch, 4
Dietrich, 91
Di Franco, 25
Dissanayake, 92
Drieschner, 9, 143-145
Duncan, 22, 135
Dowling, 4
Duras, 96

Eddington, 48
Edward, 124-129
Ely, 156, 164, 166, 167, 168
Elz, 22
Emmelkamp, 27

Forinash, 61
Freud, 82, 84, 91, 96
Frohne-Hagemann, 12, 59

Garred, 31

Gembris, 4
Gibson, 149
Gieles, 17
Gindl, 60, 150-151
Giorgi, 145, 162
Glaser, 156, 157, 162, 164
Goll, 7
Grainger, 11, 52
Gregg, 95, 96
Greimas, 81
Guba, 156, 161, 165, 167, 168
Gunderson, 23
Gustorff, 7

Haffa-Schmidt, 7
Hafkamp, 20
Hallin, 31
Hargreaves, 114
Harrer, 4
Hartogh, 90
Hayashi, 23
Heal, 73
Hegi, 12, 60, 74, 76-79
Hermans, 96
Hesse, 94
Hevner, 4
Hibben, 7
Higgins, 11
Hilliard, 154
Hillman-Boxill, 59
Horkheimer, 34
Horn, 22
Huppmann, 6
Hutschemaekers, 154

Ionesco, 45

Jensen, 23
Jochims, 59, 73
Johns, 83
Johnson, 148
Jung, 82

Kächele, 11, 60
Kapteina, 7
Kenny, 12, 31, 32, 34, 50, 52, 59, 71, 137, 181
Klee, 82
Knill, 12, 14, 59
Kraijer, 24
Krantz, 20
Krause, 135
Kristeva, 82, 92, 124

Langenberg, 11, 12, 52
Langer, 99
Lecourt, 12, 25, 59
Leff, 24
Lehtonen, 31, 60, 181
Lekanne Deprez, 155
Lerch, 135
Lewcowicz, 68
Liberman, 22
Lincoln, 156, 161, 165, 167, 168
Loos, 7, 59

Mace, 154
Mahler, G., 44
Mahler, M., 117
Mahns, 6, 7, 31, 181
Mann, 43, 44
Marshall, 153
Mastnak, 12
McNiff, 11, 52
Meltzoff, 67
Meyer, 69
Moreno, 149
Mozart, 100, 146
Mueser, 22
Mulder, 96
Müller, 7

Nattiez, 98
Newman, 148
Niedecken, 12

Nordoff-Robbins, 7, 12, 25, 123, 124-129
Nygaard Pedersen, 20, 22, 24

Odell-Miller, 16
Orlemans, 33

Pavlicevic, 11, 12, 22, 31, 59, 74, 98, 99, 102, 104, 109, 135, 181
Perilli, 22
Petersen, 26
Petzold, 7, 14
Pfeiffer, 22
Pflederer, 118
Piaget, 114, 115
Pioch, 9
Polanyi, 51
Priebe, 153
Priestley, 12, 82, 100
Puhr, 173-178

Raith, 73, 135
Ravel, 147
Rebergen, 16
Reinecke, 4
Renz, 7
Richards, 147-148
Rider, 118
Rilke, 45
Robarts, 7
Rogers, 7
Rolling Stones, 146-148
Rolvsjord, 124
Rutten-Saris, 79
Rutter, 26
Ruud, 6, 31, 181

Sackett, 154
Salber, 97
Sartre, 34
Scarlatti, 146
Schalkwijk, 6, 9, 18
Schapira, 16
Scheytt-Hölzer, 60
Schön, 13, 158
Schopler, 26
Schubert, 147
Schulz, 25
Schumacher, 7, 25, 74, 75, 76-79, 124
Schumann, 52, 147
Schwabe, 6, 9, 12
Schwandt, 156
Sechrest, 118
Seligman, 153
Serafine, 118
Shapiro, 148
Silverman, 23
Slade, 153
Sloboda, A., 7
Sloboda, J., 4
Smaling, 156
Smeijsters, 6, 7, 8, 9, 11, 12, 14, 22, 26, 44, 69, 74, 100, 104, 107, 129-133, 135, 136-143, 145-149, 153, 157, 161, 163
Smitskamp, 14
Spitzer, 4
Steen-Moeller, 16
Steinberg, 73, 135
Steiner, G., 43, 45, 46, 47
Steiner, R. 90
Stern, 12, 46, 61, 67-81, 90, 92, 98, 99, 103, 104, 111, 113-117, 120, 122, 124, 129, 134, 145, 181
Stige, 31, 32, 180, 181
Storm, 74, 100, 135, 139-141
Stratton, 4
Strauss, 57, 61, 156, 157, 162, 163, 164, 165, 168
Strobel, 6, 7, 12, 23
Summer, 90

Tang, 22
Tesch, 168
Te Velde, 14
Thoomes-Vreugdenhill, 27
Thürlemann, 82
Timmermann, 60
Tissen, 155
Trevarthen, 22, 135
Tüpker, 11, 12, 59, 62, 97, 165, 166
Turkewitz, 68
Turpin, 154

Van Audenhove, 28
Van den Berk, 16, 74, 129-130, 135
Van den Bosch, 23
Van den Hurk, 74, 100, 104, 107, 131-133, 135, 136-139, 141-143
Van der Klis, 28
Van der Poel, 20, 141
Van Engeland, 26
Van Gogh, 43
Van Laarhoven, 17
Van Loon, 25
Van Nieuwenhuijzen, 16
Vaughn, 24
Verhey, 25, 29
Verlaine, 43
Von Moreau, 7
Vroegop-Speelman, 25

Warwick, 25
Wasylenki, 22
Weber, 25
Weymann, 12, 31, 181, 185
Wheeler, 9, 11, 18, 161, 165
Whitehead, 48
Wigram, 7, 153
Wilber, 48, 49, 52
Willms, 7
Wils, 14
Wittgenstein, 32, 53, 185
Wohler, 59
Wolberg, 9
Wölfl, 7
Wunderlich, 22

Yang, 23
Yao, 22
Yin, 165, 166, 168

Zalanowski, 4
Zheng, 22

SUBJECTS

Abuse, 135
Action, 84
Active music therapy, 183
Aesthetics, 65, 71, 72, 80, 81
Aloneness, 78
Analogy, 11, 55-64, 70, 81, 84, 165, 181-182
- definition, 87-109
- in clinical practice, 135-151
- in diagnosis, 87
- in treatment, 87
- nonspecific, 87, 101, 140
- of musical interaction and independent Self, 87-134
- research, , 135-150, 168-180
- specific, 87, 101, 140

Anger, 143-145, 150
Anhedonia, 77
Anorexia nervosa, 138-139, 150-151
Anthroposophy, 63, 90
Anxiety, 26-27, 76
Apathy, 150
Art, 81-83
Arts therapies, 13, 15, 84
Assertiveness, 146-149
Assessment, 19
Assessment scales, 22-27
Association, 99, 185
Attachment, 75
Attunement, 25, 71, 76, 121, 150
Autism, 24-26, 71, 75, 121, 122, 124

Behavior
- problem, 26-27
- disturbance, 139-141

Behaviorism 27, 33, 57, 83
Blues, 72, 148-149
Body awareness, 75
Burnout, 145-149

Catatonia, 77
Categorical affects, 98
Classical music, 71, 72
Client centered, 28-29
Clinical
- experience, 154, 155-160
- practice, 135-151
- reasoning, 13
- techniques, 103, 120
  - destabilizing, 143
  - elicitation, 137
  - grounding, 143
  - imitating, 120
  - intensifying, 143
  - making spaces, 139
  - pacing, 122
  - redirection, 137, 143
  - reflecting, 123

Cognitive processing, 44-45, 92, 95, 96, 99
Cognitive therapy, 146
Coma, 75
Communication, 74, 135
Compulsion, 73, 74, 80, 135, 136-138
Conditioning, 99
Conservation and variation,
- in music, 117-119
- in music therapy, 119-124
  - sequential (Edward), 124-129
  - synchronous (Ingrid), 131-133
- music compared to language, 129-130
- psychological, 114

Coping behavior, 74
Core category, 55-64, 87-109, 182

Creativity, 61

Delusion, 117
Denial, 79
Depersonalization, 77, 117
Depression, 73, 80, 81, 135, 141, 146-149, 150
Derealization, 77, 117
Developmental psychology, 4, 63, 67-81
Diagnosis, 6
Displacement, 78
Dissociation, 77, 117
DSM-IV, 135
Dynamic form, 104

Eating disorders, 75
Education, 158-160
Embodied meaning, 69, 88
Empathy, 62, 69, 120, 123
Enuresis,, 139
Essentialism, 28
Existential-humanistic, 38
Expressed emotion, 24
Expression, 62, 185
Expressive therapy, 63

Fehlleistung, 141
Felt sense, 84
Field of play, 88, 137
Forensic psychiatry, 143-145
Form
- aesthetic, 109
- ambiguity, 95
- and content, 43-44, 81
- biological, 97
- isomorphism, 96, 97, 181
- musical, 81, 83, 88, 89, 104, 105-107, 109, 111, 116
- of feeling, 65-85, 88, 180
- of perception, 65-85

Form (continued)
- psychological, 71, 105-107, 109

Fragmentation, 77
Frustration tolerance, 74
Fugue
- musical, 96
- psychological, 77, 117

Fusion, 77, 117

Gestalt psychology and Gestalt laws, 69, 111, 118, 119
Gestalt therapy, 63
Goals, 8, 18
Grief, 105-107
Grounded theory, 57-58, 136, 162, 164
Guided Imagery and Music, 72, 95, 100

Handicap
- brain injured, 73
- mental, 71, 122

Hermeneutics, 80, 136
Holism, 28
Homology, 90, 181
Humanistic psychology, 57, 63, 83
Hysterical paralysis, 77

Icon, 98
Identity, 74, 105-107, 108
- false, 108
- personal, 133, 136, 141-143

Imitation, 125-128
Impression, 185
Improvisation Assessment Profiles, 102
Index, 98, 99
Indication, 7, 15-29, 108
Individuation, 108
Inferiority, 66
Initiation, 125-128

Integrative therapy, 63
Intermediary
- object, 45
- space, 71

Jazz, 71, 72

Knowledge
- abstract, 161
- art-based, 67, 69
- body of, 14, 155
- consensus based, 14, 29, 154
- constructed, 57, 165-166, 177, 182
- development, 155-160
- direct-indirect, 48, 51, 84, 183, 185
- evidence based, 15, 29, 154
- immediate, 32
- implicit, 70-71
- interpretational, 44, 88, 92, 102, 103
- intimate, 48, 50-53, 88, 96
- intrinsic, 101
- irrational, 45-46
- metaphoric, 48, 90, 92, 93, 95, 169, 183
- numinous, 45-46
- primary-secondary, 44-45
- sensational, 51
- symbolic, 48-50, 62, 68, 69, 81-82, 84, 88, 92, 98, 125, 139, 169, 182, 183
- tacit, 29, 99, 154, 159

Language, 6, 35
- analogous, 104
- intermediary, 101-104, 105-107
- psychological, 105
- verbal, 184-185

Learning
- competencies, 155, 158
- disabilities, 76
- double-loop, 155-160
- organization, 159-160
- self-regulated, 159-160

Legitimization, 5, 10, 12
Lifestyle, 111

Making special, 35, 38
Medicine, 100
Medium-oriented approach, 5
Morphology, 57, 63, 97, 103, 104
- Gestalt factors, 97, 98
- of feelings, 99

Mother and child interaction, 113-117
- choreography, 134
- orchestration, 134

Musical
- ability, 72,
- aesthetics, 183-184
- analysis, 102, 183
- experience, 33
- improvisation, 71, 79, 100, 104, 184
- interaction, 76, 111-134
- meaning, 183-184
- preference, 72

Multidisciplinary teams, 29
Music neurology, 4
Musicogenic epilepsy, 129
Music psychology, 4
Mystery, 34, 90

Neurological disturbances, 75
Neurology, 4, 19
Novel, 44, 96

Octave, 96, 96
Ostinato, 95, 96, 183

Paranoia, 77
Perception
 amodal, 67-68, 181, 182, 183
 cross-modal, 67-68, 185
Personality disorders, 74, 78, 81
Phenomenology, 80, 136, 145, 162
Physical doctor, 83
Polyphony, 132-133
Pop/rock, 71, 72
Preconscious, 45
Projection, 139
Protonarrative envelope, 70, 81, 89, 93, 96, 101, 149
Psychiatry, 4, 19
Psychoanalysis, 57, 63, 83, 146
Psychology, 4, 19, 55, 102
Psychology of the medium, 13, 180
Psychopathology, 102
Psychosis, 75, 77, 117
Psychosomatic disturbances, 75
Psychotherapy, 4, 83, 102
Pythagorean School, 90

Rapprochement, 138
Rationalization, 79, 141
Receptive music therapy, 65, 100, 183
Recognition, 99
Re-creating, 37
Re-exploring, 37
Referential meaning, 46-47
Reflective practitioner, 13, 21, 158, 159
Repeating, 37
Replica, 88, 91
Representation, 91, 98, 99
 analogous, 49
 injunctive, 49
 negative, 49
 semirepresentation, 91
Repression, 79, 137
Research
 category, 163-164, 171
 chain of evidence, 162, 166
 confirmability, 162, 165, 167
 constructivist, 165-166, 177
 content analysis, 172
 corroboration, 136, 145
 credibility, 105, 162, 165, 167
 data process techniques, 157-158
 dependability, 162, 165, 167
 dialogue, 166
 efficacy, 10
 experimental, 154, 161
 feedback, 167
 generalization, 161
 hypothesis-generating, 161-162
 inquiry techniques, 157-158
 intersubject, 154
 intrasubject, 154
 measuring instruments, 162
 member checking, 105, 109, 136, 145, 162, 167, 169, 170, 177, 180
 memos, 166
 methods, 9, 32
 motif
  musical, 164-165, 179
  psychological, 164, 172-175, 179
 naturalistic, 136, 155-180
 observation report, 163
 openness, 162
 panel, 170
 pattern matching, 162, 165
 peer debriefing, 14, 36, 105, 136, 162, 167, 169, 172, 177, 180
 positivism, 35, 36

Research (continued)
- qualitative, 9, 10, 33, 48, 55, 56-58, 135-143, 153, 161-162
- quantitative, 143-145, 153
- randomized controlled trials, 153
- reductionism, 10
- repeated analysis, 105, 169
- repeated observation, 162
- replication, 161
- sampling, 161
- self-report, 163
- sensitizing concept, 164, 172
- single-case, 154, 161-162
- standardization, 35
- subjectivity, 10, 162, 163, 166, 170
- thick description, 162
- time-series, 180
- topics, 4
- transcript, 163
- transferability, 136, 162, 165
- triangulation, 6, 21, 105, 109, 136, 155-160, 162, 167-168, 169
- trustworthiness, 136, 145, 162

Re-sounding, 37
Rett-syndrome, 75

Schizophrenia, 21-23, 81, 121, 135
Science, 35
Self
- core Self, 75, 76-77, 113 117,
  - Self-affectivity, 77, 113
  - Self-agency, 76, 113
  - Self-coherence, 77, 113
  - Self-history, 77, 113
  - Self-regulating experiences, 78
  - Self-regulating other, 78
- emergent Self, 75, 76
  - cross-modality, 76, 123
  - vitality affects, 76
- false Self, 78
- independent Self, 111-134
- invariants, 134
- prenatal Self, 75
- self-esteem, 131, 141
- structure of the Self, 83
- subjective Self, 75, 78-79
  - affect attunement, 78
  - sharing affection, 78
  - sharing attention, 78
  - sharing intentions, 78
- true Self, 151
- verbal self, 79
  - language, 79
  - objective Self, 79
  - symbolic play, 78

Semiotic theory, 81-82, 104, 125
- analogizing, 81
- homology, 81
- semiotic system, 81, 95
- semisymbolic system, 81, 82, 88, 94
- sign, 82, 183
- symbolic system, 81, 82

Sonata, 183
Sound healing, 65
Sounding, 37, 65, 66, 72, 81
Sound therapy, 65
Splitting, 78
Stereotyped behavior, 24-26
Structure, 62
Subconscious, 45
Symbiosis, 117

Technical, 38
Theme and variation (mother and child), 113-117
Theory, 11, 19, 31-40, 55-56, 81

Therapeutic relationship, 37
Tonmalerei, 91, 98
Transactional analysis, 146
Transitional objects, 78
Transference, 62, 146
Traumarbeit, 96
Treatment modality, 18, 22-27
Trugschluß, 112
Type A behavior, 97

Unconscious, 45, 84
Uniqueness, 34

Violence, 144
Vitality affects, 12, 67-71, 88, 98, 111, 122, 139, 144, 147, 148, 149
Vulnerability, 146, 147

Words, 43-53, 83-85, 185

THE AUTHOR

Professor Henk Smeijsters, Ph.D., is associate professor and head of research of KenVaK (Kenniskring Kennisontwikkeling Vaktherapieën), an expertise center for the arts therapies (drama therapy, music therapy, art therapy and dance-movement therapy). KenVaK is a joint venture of Zuyd University, Utrecht University, and Saxion University Enschede. Henk Smeijsters is head of studies of the master training program for arts therapies at Zuyd University, and guest professor of the Ph.D. program at Aalborg University.

Since 1980 Henk Smeijsters has been working as a researcher in music therapy. Since 1997, besides music therapy, his research includes the other arts therapies. Till 1997 he has lectured at the University of Nijmegen, the University of Professional Education Nijmegen, and the University of Professional Education Enschede. At the same time he was head of research at the Music Therapy Laboratory of the University of Professional Education Nijmegen. Between 1997 and 2002 he has been head of studies of the bachelor training programs for arts therapies at the University of Professional Education Limburg. Henk Smeijsters publishes and lectures all over the world. He is the European Editor of The Arts in Psychotherapy and a member of the Advisory Board of the Musiktherapeutische Umschau. Henk Smeijsters is a honorary member of the Dutch Association for Creative Therapy.

KenVaK started as a research center in January 2003. By means of consensus based and evidence based naturalistic research, KenVaK develops the body of knowledge of the arts therapies. KenVaK also develops bachelor and master training research programs. There is a close cooperation between the researchers of KenVaK, the association, arts therapists in The Netherlands and research centers and training institutions in Europe and the United States.